Dr Peter Miller is the director of the Hilton Head Health Institute on Hilton Head Island, South Carolina. Under his leadership the Institute has developed a widespread reputation in the fields of weight control and health promotion.

Dr Miller received his BA from the University of Maryland and his PhD in Clinical Psychology from the University of South Carolina. He has written four books and over sixty research articles on health and behaviour and is editor-in-chief of *Addictive Behaviors*, an international journal publishing studies on obesity, smoking, problem drinking and drug abuse.

D1742336

DR PETER M. MILLER

The Change Your Metabolism Diet

PANTHER
Granada Publishing

Panther Books
Granada Publishing Ltd
8 Grafton Street, London W1X 3LA

Published by Panther Books 1985

First published in the USA under the title
The Hilton Head Metabolism Diet by
Warner Books, Inc. 1983

Copyright © Peter M. Miller 1983

ISBN 0-586-06154-1

Printed and bound in Great Britain by
Collins, Glasgow

Set in Times

To Melanie and Michael

Contents

1
It's Not Your Fault

If you have tried every new diet developed over the past few years, only to gain all lost weight back again, you are definitely not alone. In fact, you're the rule rather than the exception. Over 90 per cent of people who go on diets are unsuccessful and must continue to fight the battle of the bulge. Conventional diets simply don't work.

Your failures are not your fault. You've just been going about it the wrong way. Forget everything you've ever learned about dieting. I'm going to give you a system of weight control that *does* work. My system, the Hilton Head Metabolism Diet, is the *only* permanent way to shed excess pounds and keep them off for ever. I'm not just talking about another diet, but a totally new frame of reference. Your weight problem is not due to the number of calories you eat. It's a function of how many calories you burn up.

How the Hilton Head Metabolism Diet Was Created

As a specialist in weight reduction for many years, I became frustrated by the failure of many patients to lose weight. Some would stick strictly to a diet but still prove unable to lose much weight. Others would lose but quickly regain that lost weight within two or three months. It amazed me how people on exactly the same diet and exercise programme could differ so much in the results they achieved.

To find a new approach I began listening more closely to my patients' complaints.

My friend Sally eats anything she wants and never gains an ounce. I can gain six pounds over a holiday weekend.

But, Doctor, even when I do lose weight, it's a constant struggle to keep from gaining it back. Slim people don't seem to have the same problem.

I just can't lose weight as easily as other people. Maybe it's my thyroid.

Like many of my colleagues, I used to assure these patients that their problem was not glandular. They simply ate too much. I might even have suspected a complaining patient of only making excuses for cheating on the diet.

Luckily, after a while I began to pay more attention to these complaints. I took them more seriously and began to investigate individual differences in the ability to control weight. I started by examining the records of my patients over the previous six years, comparing their eating, exercise, and weight patterns with those of slim people. Next I compiled the results of every major research study comparing weight regulation, eating, exercise, and metabolism in overweight and non-overweight individuals. To my amazement some of the most revealing research studies were to be found in very obscure medical journals. Perhaps this is why no one had connected the pieces of the weight control puzzle before.

As a result of these investigations, I radically departed from traditional ideas about dieting. I'm now very pleased that I did, because the programme I eventually developed offers a *final* solution to weight control problems.

The evidence in favour of the Hilton Head Metabolism Diet is astounding. It's been there all along. Regular or fad diets do not work, because overeating is *not* your main problem. You are overweight because of your failure to burn calories efficiently through metabolism. In most cases your metabolism is not abnormal, just sluggish.

Every major study on metabolism in the last ten years verifies this fact: the efficiency of your metabolism, although influenced by many factors, is still under your control.

The Hilton Head Metabolism Diet is designed not merely to help you lose weight, but also to enable you to change your body chemistry so that weight control becomes easier. (I will explain why you don't burn as many calories as a slim person and what you can do about it.)

You Were Right All Along

Stop feeling guilty and frustrated. Your difficulty in regulating your weight is not due to lack of willpower, laziness, or gluttony. You were right all along. You *do* gain weight more easily than slim people. I realize you've been telling people this for years and that they haven't been listening to you. Well, I believe you, and I have evidence to prove the 'experts' are wrong and you are right. Your burden of carrying all that extra weight and taking the blame for it is over.

I don't want you ever to feel guilty again or let anyone else make you feel guilty about your weight. Doctors, spouses, and friends simply don't understand, especially if they're slim. They have old-fashioned ideas about your weight. Don't accept their criticisms any more. I'm going to liberate you from all this frustration and free you from the dieting merry-go-round for the rest of your life.

A Totally New Approach

Once you begin my plan you'll realize you've finally found a totally different approach to controlling your weight. It's like discovering a medicine that has just been developed to cure your chronic disease. Most of my patients become so enthusiastic about my programme that they refer to themselves as disciples of the new 'diet breakthrough'. They can't stop talking about it.

You, too, will realize that *only* this approach to weight reduction

- Stimulates your ability to burn fat by naturally increasing your metabolic rate.

- Tunes your metabolic engine so that you burn more calories without added effort.

- Encourages you to eat *more* meals rather than less.

- Gives you four easy-to-prepare, well-balanced daily meals that completely satisfy your appetite.

- Allows you to vary your calories from week to week and thus avoid feelings of food deprivation and dietary boredom.

- Provides you with a simple, easy-to-follow exercise plan that fits easily into your day-to-day routine.

- Changes your body composition so you become firm, trim, and less flabby.

- Changes your body chemistry so, once you lose weight, you can eat normally and never gain weight again.

It Really Works

The Hilton Head Metabolism Diet not only makes sense, it really works. I see it work almost every day. It has helped my patients lose weight quickly and, more importantly, keep that weight off for ever. Patients with long histories of weight problems have been able to forget permanently about dieting. They have lost weight and now can eat normally without fear of gaining it back. By following my plan, they have successfully altered their metabolism so they burn hundreds more calories each day.

This is not a fly-by-night or fad programme. The Hilton Head Metabolism Diet is based on sound theories and has been tested on people just like you. Many of these were people who had given up on ever being able to maintain an ideal weight. It worked for them, and it will work for you, too.

My patients, who come from almost every state in the United States and several foreign countries, have learned to live normal, slim lives. A life without deprivation. A life without diets.

The Hilton Head Metabolism Diet works whether you are 10 pounds overweight or 100 pounds overweight. My records indicate that patients who follow my plan carefully *are* successful. They are maintaining a slim, ideal weight, in many cases for the first time in their lives. Those who have tried the hardest on other diets, only to fail, are my biggest successes. They have finally turned themselves into slim people for ever.

2

The Mystery of Metabolism

The first widespread notion I attacked in developing my plan was that people are overweight because they eat too much. This idea is at the very heart of every diet available. So-called 'experts' think that fat people eat too much because of gluttony, emotional problems, oral needs, or lack of willpower. To this I say, 'Nonsense!'

My first rule for you to remember is

FAT PEOPLE DO NOT

EAT MORE THAN

SLIM PEOPLE.

I don't make this statement lightly. An overwhelming number of recent studies support my view. Of course, you might eat ravenously some of the time, but so do slim people. The number of calories you eat cannot account for the difference between your weight and that of a slim friend.

If overeating were the major problem then, other factors being equal, two people eating the same low calorie diet should lose about the same amount of weight. As your own experience tells you, this just doesn't happen. Several months ago I saw two nearly identical patients. Both were women in their thirties, five feet six inches tall, and weighing 140 pounds. Neither exercised, and both were very inactive. On a 700-calorie-a-day diet, one lost six pounds in three weeks, while the other lost fourteen pounds. Both were in a controlled residential programme in which dietary meals were carefully portioned out and cheating was not possible. Based on standard notions of overeating as a cause of obesity, these women should have lost the same amount of weight.

Individual differences also show up in nutritional research on overeating. In several studies people have been asked to eat two to three times their usual amount of food to see what happens to their weight. Overweight people who do this gain weight very quickly – as much as twenty pounds in two weeks. Normal-weight and slim people rarely gain more than five or six pounds.

Well, if overeating is not the problem, then what is? I can answer that in one word – metabolism.

The Missing Link: Metabolism

To understand metabolism, think of your body as a furnace. Food is the fuel that supplies energy to run the furnace. The amount of energy in the food you eat is measured in calories. So, you eat calories each day to keep your furnace running. Your furnace burns calories through a process known as metabolism.

Metabolism is simply the energy required to keep you alive. It refers to the number of calories of food energy your body burns to maintain vital functions such as heart rate, brain activity, and digestion. Even if you were in a coma and never moved a muscle, your body would need to burn calories for energy. Generally speaking, metabolism (also know as basal metabolism or resting metabolism) refers to the number of calories your body is burning at rest – when you're not moving or doing anything. Exercise and physical activity also help you burn calories.

All of this information can be expressed more simply by means of an energy equation:

$$\underset{\text{(Calories from food)}}{\textbf{INPUT}} = \underset{\substack{\text{(Calories from metabolism} \\ \text{and activity)}}}{\textbf{OUTPUT}}$$

When all the fuel that enters the body is burned up, you maintain your normal weight. Excess fuel that is not burned is stored as fat. If you don't burn all the calories you eat, you will end up with an excess amount of fat.

Since fat people don't eat more than slim people, the cause of overweight must lie in the OUTPUT side of the equation. That's exactly right. Fat people do not burn calories as efficiently as slim people.

This is my second rule for you to remember:

FAT PEOPLE DO NOT
BURN FAT AS WELL
AS SLIM PEOPLE.

Now, you may ask, is this due to problems in metabolism or a lack of physical activity? It may actually be a combination of both, but it is primarily due to insufficient burning of calories through metabolism. While many overweight people don't get enough exercise, the same can be said of many slim people. There are simply not enough differences in the physical activity levels of fat and slim people to explain weight problems.

Metabolic Suppression

Before you jump to conclusions, let me assure you there is nothing abnormal about your metabolism. Over 95 per cent of overweight people have a normal thyroid, the gland that controls the number of calories your body burns to keep you alive. Rushing to your doctor to get thyroid hormones won't help. In fact, as I will describe later, taking these supplements when you don't need them will do your metabolism more harm than good.

While your metabolism is not abnormal, it definitely is sluggish and inefficient. You suffer from what I call *metabolic suppression*.

To understand this concept, let's go back to the idea of your body being like a furnace. Everyone has a basic, standard level at which he or she burns fuel. This basal metabolism for women is between 1200 and 1500 calories each day – that many calories are burned each day to sustain life. Men have a higher basal metabolism, ranging from 1600 to 1900 calories per day.

In addition to this base level, your rate of burning calories fluctuates throughout the day depending on various conditions. For example, your basal metabolism is stimulated when you eat, when the climate changes, and when you exercise. It's like a thermostat turning up the furnace automatically in response to fuel coming in, any drop in temperature, and increased energy demand. If your thermostat is working properly, you have a highly efficient metabolism. Your base rate of, say, 1400 calories will be stimulated several times throughout the day, and you will burn off an extra 400 to 500 calories during each twenty-four-hour period.

People suffering from metabolic suppression often have two problems. First, they are usually at the lower end of the average range of basal metabolism. Second, and even more crucial, their thermostats are defective. Not only are they burning minimal calories but also they do not have the periodic increases in metabolic rate throughout the day. The furnace does not respond to stimulation. It simply stays at a low level, regardless of changes in the body or in the environment.

Because of metabolic suppression, a woman could have a base level of only 1100 calories per day and show but very slight increases in metabolism, from 50 to 100 calories, during the day. The result could be disastrous. As many as 500 calories of food per day would not be burned off as it should be. That may not seem like a lot, but it add up to 3500 calories per week, 15,000 calories per month, and 182,500 per year. You gain one pound of fat every time your body fails to burn an extra 3500 calories. That mean you would gain one pound each week, four or five pounds each month, and over fifty pounds in a year! The slim person with an efficient metabolism can eat the same number of calories as yourself and not gain an ounce.

Don't get discouraged. I'm going to show you how to change your metabolism, to fix your thermostat so that you burn more calories. You *can* do it as long as you follow my plan. Once your body chemistry has been improved, once you release your metabolism to do what it was intended to do, you'll never have a weight problem again. Just think, you'll be like all those slim friends of yours. People will be looking enviously at *you* and saying, 'You're one of those naturally slim people. You can eat anything you want and never gain weight.'

Now that you know what your problem is, you might be wondering why you have metabolic suppression.

Why Your Thermostat is Defective

There are five basic reasons why you don't burn calories as efficiently as a slim person:

1. WHO AND WHAT YOU ARE

The ability of your body to burn calories efficiently is, in part, determined by who and what you are. First of all, your heredity is important. A tendency to gain weight easily runs in families. If one of your parents is fat, you stand a 40 per cent chance of being fat, too. If both parents are overweight, there is an 80 per cent chance you will be fat. (Identical twins who have been raised apart by families with *different* eating habits tend to weigh about the *same* as each other when they are adults.) Children of overweight parents have a lower and more sluggish metabolic rate than children of normal-weight parents. You may simply have been born with a metabolism that is not operating properly.

Other factors such as your sex and body size are also important. Generally speaking, women have a lower metabolic rate than men. People who are smaller in height and stature have a lower metabolic rate than taller, larger people. I'll go into more detail on these factors later, but for now just realize that your metabolism may be the way it is because of who your ancestors were, how tall you are, and whether you are a man or a woman. This does *not* mean that your metabolism cannot be changed. It simply points out the need for getting on my programme to change it.

2. HOW OFTEN YOU DIET

It seems strange to suggest that dieting can make your metabolism sluggish, but it's true. Whenever you reduce the number of calories you eat, your body begins to turn down its furnace. The lower the number of calories, the lower your metabolism. Your metabolic rate is reduced the most when you suddenly go on very low calorie diets or when you fast. Your body is actually fighting the weight loss process by burning fewer calories.

Why? The answer is quite simple. Our bodies are highly adaptive to change and are programmed not for dieting, but for survival. When you eat very little or stop eating altogether, your body thinks you are starving. In terms of survival, starvation can eventually lead to death. So your body concludes, 'In order to save my life I must conserve energy by burning as few calories as possible.'

3. HOW YOU EAT AND HOW YOU DIET

Inconsistent eating and dieting habits contribute to metabolic suppression. If you don't eat breakfast, or if you skip meals to lose weight, you are causing your metabolism to become more stingy about burning calories. You are working against yourself.

The very worst pattern of all is one in which periods of dieting are followed by episodes of bingeing. This is exactly what happens with most dieters. They go on a very strict diet for several days, eating as little as possible. Then they simply can't stand the deprivation anymore, so they gorge themselves for several days. Once the guilt, depression, and pounds set in, they starve themselves all over again. Sound familiar?

After many repetitions of this pattern the metabolism becomes confused. It declines with dieting and then is expected to bounce right back up quickly when you start eating again. Well, it doesn't. Instead, it rebels. It becomes sluggish and refuses to shoot back up after dieting. It stays suppressed for a much longer time, even after you're no longer dieting. As a result, when you go off your diet your metabolism is still burning very few calories. The food you eat is rapidly turned into fat. In fact, the repetition of this dieting-eating-dieting pattern over the years practically guarantees the formation of additional poundage. If you were trying to get fat and stay that way, you couldn't have chosen a better method.

4. THE DIETS YOU HAVE TRIED

Unfortunately, most of the popular diets of the last ten years not only don't help your metabolism, but contribute to its suppression. The diets that have the worse effect are the following:

- Low carbohydrate diets
- Fasts
- Liquid diets
- Protein formula diets

Let's suppose you want to lose twenty pounds. You go on one of the many popular low carbohydrate diets. Now, your body must have a sufficient amount of carbohydrates, primarily in the form of fruits, vegetables, cereal, bread, and potatoes, to supply glucose to the cells. Your cells need glucose for energy. If you're not eating enough carbohydrates to supply your glucose requirements, your body does a very logical thing. It converts the protein you are eating into carbohydrate and then into glucose. That's right. Your body has the capability of turning some nutrients into other ones. It's as though your furnace were changing coal into oil.

Now, when that happens – and it happens on *every* diet I've listed – you run into another problem. Since the protein you eat is being changed to carbohydrate, your body doesn't get enough protein to satisfy its protein needs.

In its search to provide for this need, your body turns to the most readily available alternate source of protein – muscle tissue. It simply burns muscle – your muscle – to provide the missing protein.

In the final analysis you wind up with the following weight loss:

> Water loss　=　5 pounds
> Fat loss　　= 10 pounds
> Muscle loss　=　5 pounds

You feel great because you've lost twenty pounds. If only you could look inside your body. It wasn't twenty pounds of fat lost, only ten. 'So what?' you may ask. Twenty pounds is twenty pounds.

The problem arises when you get off the diet and begin to gain those pounds back again. Once you gain back your weight, as most dieters do, the twenty pounds look like this:

> Water gain　=　5 pounds
> Fat gain　　= 15 pounds
> Muscle gain　=　0 pounds

There's your twenty pounds, all right. But look closely. That's not the same twenty pounds you started out with. The low carbohydrate diet changed your body composition. Somewhere in the process you lost five pounds of muscle and gained five pounds of fat. You're still twenty pounds overweight, but now you are *fatter* than before.

Metabolism is greatly influenced by the ratio of fat to muscle in your body. The more fat and the less muscle, the lower your metabolism. You ended up with a more sluggish metabolism after the diet, *because* of the diet. If you had gone on the right kind of dietary programme, the one I will put you on, this never would have happened. The more fad diets you've been on, the more you've suppressed your metabolism and the more you need my plan.

5. HOW ACTIVE YOU ARE

If you avoid physical activity, your metabolic rate is probably very sluggish. The right kinds of exercise stimulate your metabolism and help you burn more calories. You not only burn calories during physical activity, but for several hours afterwards your metabolism remains stimulated. When you've had a very physically active day, you actually end up with a higher metabolic rate that night while you are sleeping because of your exercise. In addition, exercise builds muscle tissue, which changes body chemistry to boost metabolism even higher.

You don't have to become a marathon runner or super athlete to accomplish these goals. I will put you on a reasonable, easy-to-follow physical activity plan that you will enjoy.

Are You a Victim of Metabolic Suppression?

Anyone who has been overweight off and on for two years or more definitely suffers from metabolic suppression. If you have doubts about your metabolism, try the following quiz which I have devised. Just answer 'Yes' or 'No' to each question.

METABOLIC SUPPRESSION TEST

	Yes	No
1. Are you more than fifteen pounds overweight?		
2. Do you frequently skip breakfast?		
3. Do you skip meals to cut down on calories?		
4. Do you frequently fluctuate between periods of dieting and periods of overeating?		
5. Have you been on any low carbohydrate diet or fast more than twice in the last two years?		
6. Do you get little or no exercise?		
7. Did either of your parents have a weight problem?		
8. Are you shorter than 5'5" if you are a woman and 5'9" if you are a man?		
9. Are you a woman?		

10. Do you have a long ———— ————
    history of unsuccessful
    dieting?

Give yourself 10 points for each 'Yes' answer and rate
yourself on the scale below.

Total Score	Extent of Metabolic Suppression
70-100	Severe
50-60	Moderate
30-40	Mild
0-20	None

If you are overweight and have a score of 30 or higher,
you definitely need my plan. If you scored 50 or higher,
don't waste a minute: start putting the metabolism plan
into practice today.

QUESTIONS AND ANSWERS

Q. *What medical tests can I take to see if I have metabolic
suppression?*
A. Metabolic suppression, as I have described it, is impossible to detect using standard clinical tests. Your
doctor measures your metabolism through a blood test
from which he determines the amount of thyroid hormone
in the bloodstream. These hormones influence the rate of
basal metabolism. The results simply tell you if your
hormones are within a normal range. A thyroid test
cannot tell you how many calories you burn each day.

The exact number of calories you burn can be determined by measuring your oxygen consumption and
carbon dioxide output. Unfortunately, the equipment
needed to make these determinations is only available at
very specialized clinics or at departments of exercise

physiology in universities. Additionally, while this equipment could measure your resting metabolic rate, it can't provide an exact determination of the efficiency of your metabolism. (Efficiency refers to the ups and downs in your metabolic rate throughout the day.)

Q. *Why has my doctor told me that there is nothing wrong with my metabolism?*

A. Because his tests probably indicate that there is nothing *abnormal* about your thyroid gland. He has no method of measuring the efficiency of your metabolism.

Q. *If something is wrong with my metabolism, shouldn't I be taking thyroid hormones?*

A. Thyroid hormones are only needed by a very small percentage of people: those who suffer from a glandular abnormality. Metabolic suppression does *not* require thyroid medication. These hormones have little effect if you don't need them. In fact, in the long run, your thyroid gland may react by doing less work.

Q. *If my metabolism is sluggish, will my heart rate and blood pressure be low?*

A. While there is a general relationship between heart rate and metabolism, heart rate is not a reliable indicator of metabolic rate. Blood pressure and metabolism are not related to one another.

Q. *My husband is a very nervous person. Does that mean he has a high metabolism?*

A. Not necessarily. Some people who are nervous have a high metabolism, and some have a low metabolism.

Q. *What diets should I avoid to keep my metabolism healthy?*

A. Just about all those that have been popular over the past ten years. You should especially avoid diets that are low in carbohydrates, very high in protein, or high in fat. Fasting, liquid diets, and diets below 700 to 800 calories should be avoided. The simplest rule to remember is to stay away from all diets except the Hilton Head Metabolism Diet.

Q. *Why hasn't someone told me all this before?*

A. Because even health professionals know very little about metabolism. Most of the best research in this area is done by a scattered handful of scientists who study metabolism but don't treat overweight patients.

3

Age, Sex, and Muscle

You might be wondering what age, sex, and muscle have in common! – they all exert a strong influence on metabolic rate. Before I put you on the Hilton Head Metabolism Diet, we must examine the question 'What makes one person's metabolism different from another's?' You might be amazed to discover that such things as how much muscle you have, what medicines you take, what kind of climate you live in, and how active you are after each meal all affect the number of calories you burn each day.

Factors that influence metabolism can be divided into three categories. First, *personal characteristics,* such as body size and age, are important. Second, *nutritional habits,* such as how and what you eat, make a difference in metabolism. Third, *external factors,* such as stress, climate, and drugs, have an influence. The following is an outline of the most important influences on your metabolism:

PERSONAL CHARACTERISTICS

1. Body size
2. Age
3. Sex
4. Muscle fat ratio

NUTRITIONAL AND EXERCISE HABITS

1. Spacing of meals
2. Nutritional balance
3. 'Thermogenesis'
4. Type and amount of exercise

EXTERNAL FACTORS

1. Stress
2. Climate
3. Drugs
4. Hormones
5. Caffeine and nicotine

In this chapter I shall focus on the characteristics of your body that determine metabolic rate.

Body Size

Generally speaking, the bigger you are the more calories you burn. It simply takes more energy to run a large furnace than a small one. Your total body size, known scientifically as your 'surface area', is based on both your height and weight.

I'll give you an actual example of the difference body size can make. Two of my patients, Barbara and Claire, are both in their mid thirties. Both have successfully lost weight and are maintaining their losses. Barbara is small in stature at five feet one inch and weighing 110 pounds. Claire is a tall woman of five feet nine inches, weighing 140 pounds (an ideal weight for her height). Because of this size difference, Barbara's basal metabolism is 1250 calories per day, while Claire's is 1500. Claire's body burns 250 more calories of energy each day just because she is bigger. That also means that, other factors being equal, Claire can eat 250 calories more than Barbara every day without gaining weight. It may not seem fair, but it's a basic rule of metabolism. The only exception to this rule is in the case of a young child. Even though children are much smaller in size than adults, they burn calories at a much higher rate. This continues until late adolescence. The reason for this higher metabolism is that the bodily processes involved in growth require a great deal of energy. When growth rate declines, so does metabolism.

All this just goes to show you that the determination of metabolism is a very individual matter. The Hilton Head Metabolism Diet will allow you to take these individual differences into account and use them to your advantage.

Age

We're all familiar with 'middle age spread'. Almost everyone has a friend or relative who was thin all his life only to develop a substantial 'spare tyre' around the middle after the age of forty. Perhaps that friend or relative is you!

As most people realize, metabolism declines with age. During adulthood the body's energy output gradually slows down. The most noticeable drop occurs during your mid forties and slowly continues for the rest of your life.

A fifty-five-year-old person burns about 100 to 150 fewer calories per day than a twenty-five-year-old. That can make a difference of ten to fifteen pounds of excess fat per year. Ten pounds a year may not seem like a lot, but over the years it can quickly add up. One day you might look in the mirror for a little physical self-analysis and find you're forty pounds overweight. Well, those forty pounds didn't appear overnight. And because of changes in metabolism with age, they could very well have developed without you eating even one calorie more than you did ten years ago. Dr Jean Mayer, the noted nutritionist, aptly refers to this age related fat condition as 'creeping obesity'.

Sex

Before you get too excited about this section, let me explain that here sex refers to your gender, not your behaviour. Unfortunately, if you are a woman, your body burns 10 to 15 per cent fewer calories each day than does a man's body. Given approximately the same body size, the metabolism of a thirty-five-year-old woman is equal to that of a sixty-five-year-old man! That is why the daily basal metabolism for men ranges between 1600 and 1900 calories, with the basal energy output for women being only 1200 to 1500 calories.

Because of this, men can generally eat more than women. They also lose weight more quickly when dieting. Women should never compare their eating patterns or weight losses with those of men. It's like comparing apples and oranges and is a very unrealistic way of looking at weight control.

Please don't get discouraged by these gender differences. They are mostly due to differences in muscle tissue between men and women. By following my system women can compensate for a large portion of this factor.

Muscle

Your body is composed of many different elements and structures, including muscle, fat, skin, bone, water, and internal organs, just to name a few. In terms of metabolism, the most essential ingredients in your body are the amounts of muscle and fat tissue you have.

Let's talk about fat for a minute. You are *supposed* to have fat in your body. Fat serves as an excellent energy source and is a great insulator. It's just that most people have too much of it. Ideally, men should have 15 to 18 per cent body fat. Women are by nature supposed to have more fat than men – between 20 and 25 per cent is considered ideal. That means that if a woman weighs 135 pounds, approximately 20 per cent of her weight or 27 pounds should be composed of fat. With that amount of body fat, a woman would look slim. Unfortunately, most women have a lot more than 20 per cent body fat. In fact, the average American woman has about 35 to 40 per cent fat. It is possible that when you are overweight, your body may be composed of as much as 50 to 60 per cent fat.

Your total weight minus your fat weight is called your 'lean body mass'. Someone with little fat and a lot of muscle, such as a professional athlete, would have a high lean body mass. Bill Rodgers, the top-ranked American running star, has only 5 per cent body fat and is made up mostly of lean mass.

If you weigh 150 pounds and your fat content is 30 per cent, your body would contain 45 pounds of fat. By subtracting 45 pounds from your weight of 150 pounds we find that your lean body mass is 105 pounds. You are 45 pounds of fat and 105 pounds of muscle, bone, and everything else.

Why is lean body mass so important? Because one of the most important facts about metabolism is that *the more muscle and the less fat you have, the higher your metabolism is*. People who have a lot of lean body mass burn many more calories per day than people who have a small amount of lean body mass.

The reason for this is that muscle tissue is metabolically more active than fat tissue. It takes more body energy for muscle to function. Fat is relatively inactive, while muscle cells are extremely active even when you are resting. A muscular furnace is constantly burning food fuel at a rapid rate day after day.

This relationship between lean body mass and metabolism is extremely important. For one thing, it explains why women have a lower metabolism than men. The main reason is because women biologically have more body fat and less muscle than men. When we compare men and women with similar fat and muscle contents, their metabolic rates are the same. That's great news for women! Your lower metabolism is not inevitable. Women should have a slightly higher fat content than men, but they can close the metabolic gap by achieving their lowest ideal fat percentage. This can be accomplished most effectively through the diet and exercise programme of the Hilton Head Metabolism Diet.

The explanation of why metabolism declines with age is the same. As people get older, their body fat increases. This seems due to the fact that as people age they become less and less physically active. If body fat and muscle tissue remain stable, there is no metabolic decline with age.

How Much Fat Do You Have?

Since your age and gender are not likely to change, a major goal of the Hilton Head Metabolism Diet is to lower your body fat and increase your lean body mass. As I mentioned in Chapter 2, some diets actually *reduce* lean body mass, causing your metabolism to drop even lower. I get so frustrated when I see people going on one fad diet after another. They couldn't be doing themselves more harm.

At the outset you may be interested in getting a good estimate of your fat and lean content. Such an estimate would determine just how badly off you are. It would also help you evaluate your progress as you lose weight on the Hilton Head Metabolism Diet. However, you cannot tell how much fat someone has simply by knowing his weight. It is possible to be at an ideal weight but still have too much body fat.

There are several ways to find out how much fat you have. Unfortunately, none is simple, and most require equipment that only universities, medical schools, or research centres have. The most accurate method is *hydrostatic* or *underwater weighing*. In this method a person is completely submerged in a special tank of water. Fat weight is determined by taking into account the average density of fat displacing the water. Fat is more buoyant in water than muscle. That's why fat people can float a lot easier than slim people.

Another popular method is the use of skinfold calipers to measure the fat directly beneath the skin. Specially made pincers are used to measure the thickness of folds of skin and fat at different parts of the body.

CALCULATING YOUR FAT/LEAN BODY WEIGHT

The easiest and most practical way for you to calculate your fat and lean is by taking your body measurements. Simply by measuring your waist and thigh and using a special mathematical formula you can work out your fat and lean percentages. (If you are easily confused by numbers or are not interested in your specific fat content, skip over this section and go on to the next chapter. You can follow the Hilton Head Metabolism Diet without knowing these exact numbers.)

Start by purchasing a good quality tape measure. Make sure it measures in inches on one side and centimetres on the other. Now take the following measurements and be sure to follow my directions carefully. Take your time and try to be as accurate as possible. It's easier if you have a friend or relative to assist you.

WAIST MEASUREMENT. This is a special waist measurement, so forget how you might have done this in the past. First, put your hands on your sides on either side of your waist and feel around for the top part of your pelvis. For many people it's about at the level of the belly button. Now wrap the tape around your waist at that level and read your measurement in centimetres, not inches. (If you only have inches on your tape measure, simply multiply the inches by 2.53 to convert to centimetres.)

THIGH MEASUREMENT. This measurement is fairly simple to obtain. Measure around your thigh at a point halfway between your knee and the top of your leg. Read the tape in centimetres, or again multiply the inches by 2.53.

To find out how much fat you have, you're going to have to do a little arithmetic based on these measurements. It shouldn't take you more than a couple of minutes by hand or using a calculator.

To calculate fat and lean body weight:

1. Multiply your waist measurement by .592.
2. Multiply your thigh measurement by .36.
3. Add these two amounts together.
4. Subtract 53.11 from this total.
5. Multiply your answer by 2.2.

This final figure is your fat weight in pounds. To find your lean body mass, simply subtract your fat weight from your total weight. To find your fat weight percentage, divide your fat weight by your total weight and multiply by 100.

C.Y.M.D.–B

Let me give you an example of how I usually do this with my patients. Veronica is a thirty-six-year-old attractive housewife with two children. At the time she began the Hilton Head Metabolism Diet she was 30 pounds overweight. At five feet seven inches tall, she weighed 163 pounds. Based on my original measurements, her waist was thirty-nine inches (99 centimetres), and her thigh was twenty-three-and-a-half inches (50 centimetres). Her fat and lean body weights as calculated using the above formula were as follows:

FAT WEIGHT	= 59 pounds
FAT PERCENTAGE	= 36 per cent
LEAN BODY WEIGHT	= 104 pounds
LEAN BODY PERCENTAGE	= 64 per cent

This indicated that the amount of fat in her body was much too high and that her lean body mass was too low. Her metabolism was definitely being suppressed. This could not have been discovered just by knowing her total body weight.

In Veronica's case her metabolism was being suppressed by 180 calories per day because of these fat and lean percentages. And this was only one of the many factors causing her metabolic problems. I could see the feeling of relief on her face as she finally found the reason for her weight problem. No more guilt, depression, or self-blame. No more feelings of being 'different' and weak-willed.

After seven weeks on the Hilton Head Metabolism Diet, Veronica had lost 30 pounds and had attained her weight goal of 133 pounds. Her fat content decreased from 36 per cent to 25 per cent, and her lean body mass increased from 64 per cent to 75 per cent. She was finally slim, trim and happy.

The most astonishing change occurred in her metabolism. Veronica's own words tell the story best: 'At one hundred and sixty-three pounds I was eating two thousand calories a day and gaining weight. After the Hilton Head Metabolism Diet, I'm thirty pounds lighter and able to eat twenty-five-hundred calories every day *without gaining an ounce*. I feel normal for the first time in fifteen years!'

4

Adding Fuel to the Fire

When you eat, *how often* you eat, and *what* you eat can help or hinder your metabolism. Your body's furnace must be able to regulate itself, to respond to changes just as the boiler in your house does. Metabolism is simply the production of heat energy by your body. Your internal thermostat regulates your metabolism in response both to the fuel (food) you eat and how often you eat it.

When you eat erratically, missing meals at times and overeating at others, your thermostat turns down your metabolism to conserve energy. When you eat the wrong kinds of food, you gradually change your body chemistry so that your energy output becomes smaller. Let's examine these changes in more detail so I can show you how to keep your thermostat at full throttle.

What Is the Best Fuel?

The three basic kinds of fuel that keep your furnace running are *proteins, carbohydrates,* and *fats.* In fact, these are the only things you eat that your body can use for energy.

Protein is essential for building and repairing body tissue. It is found primarily in such foods as eggs, milk, cheese, chicken, meat, lentils, dried beans, and nuts.

Carbohydrates are sources of long-term energy. There are two basic types: complex and simple. Complex carbohydrates are found in fruits, vegetables, potatoes, cereals, and bread. Simple carbohydrates are sugars such as those found in sweets, puddings, and soft drinks.

Fat is needed for quick energy and lubrication. Animal fats are found in such foods as butter, whole milk, and red meats. Vegetable fats are found in vegetable oil and margarine.

The *best* fuel for your metabolism is actually a special combination of these nutrients. The combination that is optimum for your metabolism is one in which your diet is made up of the following percentages of nutrients:

Protein	15 per cent
Carbohydrates	55 per cent
Fats	30 per cent

You might be surprised by these proportions, especially if you have been under the impression that protein is good for you and carbohydrates are bad. If you eat *more* protein than this, it will simply be converted into body fat. That's right! Nutrients that are not needed by your body are stored as fat. And you certainly don't need any more of that.

The typical American diet is way out of balance. Most people get about 43 per cent of their calories from fats, 42 per cent from carbohydrates (mostly sugar), and 15 per cent from protein. Actually, people in 1900 ate more as they were supposed to than we do in the 1980s. They also ate *more* – but weighed *less* than people nowadays. In those days people burned more calories by eating the proper foods, being more physically active, eating regularly scheduled meals each day, and being exposed to greater temperature extremes at home. The 'comforts' of our modern life, together with the fast-paced tempo of our day-to-day existence, have had a devastating effect on metabolism.

Two of the first foods that people eliminate when dieting are potatoes and bread. This is totally wrong. These are exactly the types of food you should continue to eat when trying to lose weight. They are excellent sources of carbohydrates, and carbohydrates are essential for metabolic efficiency.

An abundance of potatoes, bread, cereal, vegetables, and fruit are needed in your diet for two reasons.

First, carbohydrates ensure that you will lose a maximum amount of body fat and a minimum of lean body tissue. Remember (from Chaper 2), when your body doesn't get enough carbohydrate, it converts protein to carbohydrate and then becomes deficient in protein. That's when you start burning muscle instead of fat. This is probably the *worst* thing that can happen to your metabolism. Don't forget – the less muscle, the slower your metabolism.

Second, a diet high in carbohydrates helps guard against the drastic declines in metabolism that occur when you diet. When you lower calorie intake on any diet, your metabolism temporarily declines a bit. You can compensate for this decline by following the Hilton Head Metabolism Diet. Part of the aim is to keep your carbohydrate intake high. Low carbohydrate diets have the most severe effect on thyroid hormones, reducing them to very low levels during the diet and thereby reducing your metabolism.

For overall health, there are two nutrients that you must be careful of. You must eat *fewer simple carbohydrates* – sugar, sweets, soft drinks, pies, and cakes. These should make up no more than 10 per cent of your total calories per day. Excessive sugar consumption has been implicated in blood sugar problems, such as hypoglycaemia and diabetes, and in heart disease.

Animal fat should also be reduced to no more than 25 to 30 per cent of your total caloric intake. This means you should eat less red meat, processed luncheon meat, fat-containing dairy products, salad oils, and fried foods.

Don't let all of this talk about combinations of nutrients scare you. I have figured out the exact number of proteins, carbohydrates, and fats for you. There's no guesswork involved. Simply follow the diet I've outlined in Chapter 8, and you'll be on the road to maximum metabolic efficiency.

How Much Should You Eat? – A Three-Phase Approach

Ever get bored on a diet, eating the same type and amount of food day after day? Well, most people do. I routinely ask patients who have been on other diets, 'Why can't you stick with it?' Many will say, 'I just get bored with the same old diet.' Others say, 'I feel deprived. Everyone else is eating normally and I have to eat *diet* foods.' Or, 'I get tired of having to prepare special meals for myself. It takes too much effort.'

The Hilton Head Metabolism Diet is definitely different because

YOU WILL *NOT* GET BORED.

YOU WILL *NOT* FEEL DEPRIVED.

YOU WILL *NOT* EAT DIET FOOD.

This is because you'll be eating normal, everyday food that everyone else in the family can eat. And the diet includes *three* phases, and you'll be eating different amounts of food in each phase.

1. THE LOW-CAL PHASE

While some people may be able to lose weight on as much as 1200 or 1500 calories, those with metabolic suppression must reduce their calories at the beginning of the diet to about 800 calories a day. At this level you can and you *will* lose weight. I have found that this Low-cal Phase results in the optimum weight loss while still providing a good nutritional balance. (It is almost impossible to provide the daily minimum requirements of protein, carbohydrates, and fats on fewer than 700 to 800 calories a day.)

You will start off on the Low-cal Phase and continue this reduced intake of calories for the first *two weeks* of the diet. If you only have a few pounds to lose, you may need only *one week* of this phase.

2. THE BOOSTER PHASE

The Hilton Head Metabolism Diet compensates for the fact that your metabolism slows down when you drastically reduce calories. *No other diet does this.*

Remember, your body thinks you're starving, so it conserves energy by burning fewer calories. To stir up your metabolism during the diet, after two weeks you will be switching over to the Booster Phase. During this phase, you will be eating about 300 calories per day more than in the Low-cal Phase.

This is like revving up your engine every once in a while so it doesn't stall. If you have to lose twenty or more pounds, you'll spend two weeks in the Low-cal Phase and then one week in the Booster Phase. If you have more weight to lose, you'll switch back to the Low-cal Phase and keep alternating between Low-cal and Booster.

This switchover to the Booster Phase is very important.

It keeps your metabolism going strongly until we can get you back to a normal number of calories again.

You must switch to this phase when the time comes. Later, I'll tell you exactly when to make the switch, based on your individual weight loss.

3. THE REENTRY PHASE

The Reentry Phase is one of the most important elements of the Hilton Head Metabolism Diet. It bridges the gap between the diet proper and long-range maintenance.

This phase is mandatory, because your metabolism does not adjust quickly to change in your diet. If you suddenly went from 800 or 1000 calories to 2000 or 2500 calories, your metabolism would be slow to react. Ideally, your metabolism should increase to burn up the additional calories. However, unless you increase calories *gradually*, you run the risk of gaining some or all of your weight back soon after the diet is over.

You will be losing 90 per cent of the pounds you intend to lose during the diet – the Low-cal and Booster phases. The remaining 10 per cent will be lost during the Reentry Phase. Think of this as a pre-maintenance period during which you're getting your metabolism ready for normal eating again.

Reentry takes one week. During this time you will gradually be increasing your daily intake of calories from 1100 to 1500 in the Booster Phase to your maintenance level of calories. Your maintenance level is the maximum number of calories you can eat and still keep a steady weight. Because of the metabolic effect, it will be much higher than it was before your diet. (Maintenance calories vary from person to person. I'll show you how to find out what is best for you.)

How Often Should You Eat?

How many meals you eat during the day is very important to your metabolism. I'm not talking about how many calories you eat in total, but how they are spaced out. It's not just how much you eat; it's also how you eat it.

When dieting, you will lose weight more quickly if you eat several meals a day rather than only one or two meals. Of course, you must eat fewer calories to lose weight, but you lose more efficiently if you spread them out.

How many meals are best? Well, you certainly can't lead a normal life and eat twelve meals a day. It wouldn't be practical, and I'm sure you wouldn't be able to stick to a routine like that very long. I have found that *four meals a day* is the optimum number in terms of metabolism and practicality. This number promotes rapid weight loss without interfering with your life or making you a slave to food. Remember, if you want to keep a high metabolism, you'll have to continue with this meal plan for the rest of your life. Four meals a day, *every* day, will keep you slim for ever.

You will be eating *breakfast, lunch, dinner,* and, what I call the *metabo-meal.* As you'll see, the metabo-meal is like a light, late-night supper.

The importance of the number of meals you eat was clearly demonstrated by British scientists in a now classic nutritional study. A group of students was fed an extra 1800 calories per day for several weeks to see how much weight they would gain. Some were given their 1800 calories all in one meal. Others were given it in small portions throughout the day, about 100 calories each hour. Even though all the students were eating exactly the same number of extra calories, the 'one meal' students gained considerably more weight than the students receiving numerous small meals. Somehow the students eating many smaller meals were able to burn up more of their food calories. How was this possible? Actually, it is quite simple. It was the result of a common metabolic process that has been recognized since the 1920s.

ADDING FUEL TO THE FIRE

Without realizing it, these students were experiencing *dietary thermogenesis*, or more simply, the *thermic effect*. Whenever you eat, your body begins to burn more calories because of the energy needed to digest and absorb the food. Your furnace is charged up to burn the extra fuel that's coming in.

It was once thought that only protein foods stimulated the metabolism. We now know that carbohydrates and fats also have this effect. However, protein does require the most bodily energy to be broken down and assimilated.

The thermic effect is extremely significant for controlling your weight. After a meal your metabolism increases between 10 and 35 per cent. It remains stimulated for the next two to three hours. The more meals you eat, the more your metabolism is stimulated. With a thermic effect of 20 per cent you could be burning an extra 25 calories after each meal. By eating four meals a day you would be burning an extra 100 calories daily without even trying.

I've heard patients say, 'But I nibble all day long. Why doesn't the thermic effect keep me thin?' It's because I'm talking about metabolic responses to *meals*, not to little snacks here and there. The thermic effect is only stimulated by a meal-size quantity of food. Many people who are overweight nibble in the late afternoon and evening, but they also skip breakfast and lunch. That's why they nibble.

Fat people are at a distinct disadvantage when it comes to the thermic effect. That's because they suffer from *metabolic suppression*. Their thermic effect is very, very small. The average increase in metabolism after a meal is 26 per cent for someone who is lean with little body fat. Fat people usually show an increase of only 9 per cent, and in some cases it is as low as 3 per cent. Being fat suppresses this natural process of the body just when you need it the most. This problem can be critical. It can account for about 70 calories a day that you're not burning properly.

All this means that you *must* lower your body fat and you *must* eat four regular meals every day. A little later I'll go into more detail on when you should eat and how you should space your meals.

5

We're Not Finished Yet

Believe it or not, there are a lot more factors that influence metabolism. Let's see if there might be other ways you could be suppressing yours. You must get control of as many of these factors as possible to achieve the needed impact.

After-effects of Exercise

I'm sure you're aware that you burn more calories when you exercise. Did you know that, long after you have finished exercising, this physical activity is still having an effect on your resting metabolism? It's like the thermic effect after eating.

For several hours *after* a brisk or lengthy walk, jog, swim, or bicycle ride, your metabolism is higher than it was before the exercise. Let's suppose you shovel snow from your driveway and pavement between five o'clock and six o'clock one evening. It is strenuous work, and you really feel like you've had a workout. As a result of shovelling, your metabolism during the early hours of sleep that night would be 10 to 15 per cent higher than normal.

I will put you on a moderate, consistent exercise plan that will stimulate your metabolism and keep it stimulated. The secret is in the *timing* of your exercise, not in its intensity. Physical activity, spaced out at proper intervals twice daily, can keep the exercise-thermic effect going day after day.

Climate

Air temperatures can have a marked effect on metabolism. It is well known that extremes of heat or cold increase your metabolic rate. The resting metabolism of people who live in a hot, tropical climate or cold, arctic climate is about 5 to 10 per cent higher than that of people living in a moderate climate. Even in moderate climates, your metabolism increases whenever you are exposed to cold (below 50°F) or hot (about 90°F) temperatures for any length of time. If you've ever had to stand out in 20°F weather watching the local Armistice Day parade, at least you have the satisfaction of knowing that you were burning more calories than normal.

As part of their metabolic suppression problem, fat people do not get the same metabolic benefits from climate as their lean friends. This is especially true in cold weather. Since body fat is such a great insulator, fat people do not have the metabolic increases in cold weather that slim people do. Don't worry. As you lose body fat and increase lean body mass on the Hilton Head Metabolism Diet, you will begin to respond normally to temperature extremes.

What else can you do? Well, I won't suggest that you move to the Sahara Desert or the North Pole. You *must*, however, get yourself used to a different temperature environment. The recent energy crisis, necessitating slightly less comfortable thermostat settings in homes and public buildings, has done wonders for the country's collective metabolism.

Keep your home thermostat settings at 68°F in the winter. If you gradually get used to temperature extremes, this change won't bother you very much but will acclimatize you better to extremes of outside temperatures.

All in all, although the metabolic benefits from these changes are small compared to other elements of the Hilton Head Metabolism Diet plan, every little bit helps. A few more calories burnt daily here and there can take care of several excess pounds per year. Remember, *more* calories burned means *more* calories to eat.

Stress

Being under stress or feeling emotionally upset has an influence on metabolic rate. Some studies have found as much as a 20 per cent increase in resting metabolism due to stressful life events. This stimulation of energy output is due to increases in heart rate, adrenalin output, and muscle tension during stress reactions.

Don't worry. I'm not going to suggest you purposefully keep yourself anxious and tense all the time. The overall effect of stress on most people's metabolism is quite small. Just be aware of this effect, and don't be so quick to take tranquillizers to cope with stress.

Drugs

While most drugs have little or no effect on metabolic rate, others seem to have a noticeable impact. Research is scanty in this area, and some of these effects are still speculative. We know, for example, that people taking antidepressant medications often put on weight more easily, and it is suspected that these prescriptions slow down metabolism. Women taking female hormones in the form of birth control pills or as supplements during the menopause find themselves more likely to gain weight than before they started taking the hormone. These supplements may very well be affecting metabolism.

However, you should never discontinue the use of any medication just because you think it is interfering with your metabolism. You may need that medication for other reasons. Always consult your doctor if you have any worries in that area.

Caffeine and Nicotine

Caffeine from coffee or tea and nicotine from cigarettes have a slight stimulating effect on metabolism. This may be one reason why smokers who give up sometimes gain weight. Their metabolic rates have been artificially stimulated by the nicotine, and without cigarettes, the body must adjust to a new level. The overall changes in metabolism due to nicotine and caffeine intake are small, especially compared to those resulting from exercise or the thermic effect after meals. Also, the health risks of excessive intake of these substances would outweigh any potential usefulness they have for metabolic stimulation.

6

More Questions and Answers about Metabolism

Here are some of the most typical questions patients ask me about metabolism:

Q. *When you say I have to reduce my body fat do you mean that I should have fewer fat cells?*

A. No. As you lose weight, the fat cells you have will shrink in size. You cannot diminish the number of these cells, only their size. The number, in fact, may be genetically determined or may be determined by a combination of heredity and eating patterns in infancy. According to the 'fat cell theory', some people may be born with more fat cells than others and, because of this, gain weight more easily.

Q. *I'd like to stimulate my metabolism by developing more lean body mass, but I don't want to be overly muscular or musclebound.*

A. Don't worry. I don't want you to be overly muscular either. The kind of exercises I'll prescribe will firm and tone your muscles. You will look slim, trim, and lean, not musclebound.

Q. *I used to be very athletic when I was younger. I was very firm and muscular. Did I gain weight because my muscles turned to fat and slowed down my metabolism?*

A. Muscle cannot turn into fat. Muscle cells are muscle cells, and fat cells are fat cells. As you get older and are less active, your fat cells grow in size and your muscle cells diminish in size from lack of use.

Q. *I drink a lot of coffee and smoke about a packet of cigarettes every day. If caffeine and nicotine stimulate my metabolism, how come I'm twenty pounds overweight?*

A. Coffee drinking and cigarette smoking are only two factors that affect metabolism. They happen to be minor factors and, by themselves, account for a very slight metabolic stimulation that is negligible compared to other factors. Also, nicotine is so harmful to your health that it should never be used to stimulate metabolism. In fact, cigarette smoking is much more detrimental to overall health than being overweight is.

Q. *If high temperatures stimulate metabolism, do you recommend thermal exercise suits to increase body temperature doing exercise?*

A. Definitely not. These plastic suits do not stimulate metabolic rate and do not significantly increase body temperature. They are a waste of time and money.

Q. *I've recently read about brown fat and metabolism in a magazine article. What is brown fat and how does it affect me?*

A. Brown fat (brown adipose tissue) is a special type of fat tissue located in the upper neck and back area. This tissue is found in greatest abundance in newborn infants, small mammals living in cold climates, and animals that hibernate. Some scientist believe this tissue helps to regulate metabolism. They theorize that biochemical activity in this tissue decreases metabolic rate to help animals survive during long periods of hibernation. The exact significance of brown fat in human metabolism is still under study.

Q. *I've been taking HCG injections to lose weight. Do these injections stimulate my metabolism?*

A. Definitely not. HCG injections are one of the biggest hoaxes in the treatment of weight control. HCG stands for human chorionic gonadotropin, a hormone found in the urine of pregnant women. These injections were originally developed by two British physicians in Italy and are supposed to help your body burn fat at a faster rate. Every study of these injections has found them to be completely worthless for weight control. They have no effect on your metabolism. The 500-calorie diet that accompanies the injections may actually worsen your metabolic suppression problem.

Q. *My doctor told me not to go on any diet below 1000 calories. Does that mean that I can't go on the Hilton Head Metabolism Diet?*

A. Your doctor is probably worried that you won't get an adequate nutritional balance under 1000 calories per day. The Hilton Head Metabolism Diet is very well balanced and, therefore, is healthy for you. Also, you're eating less than 1000 calories for only two weeks at a time. Show your doctor this book and ask him to look over the diet. Of course, you should never go on any diet without your physician's approval, since only he knows your medical history and current state of health.

Q. *I've heard that muscle weighs more than fat. If I lose fat but gain muscle tissue, won't I be defeating my purpose?*

A. No. Although muscle does weigh more than fat, you must decrease fat and increase muscle to speed up your metabolism. You will still lose weight. In fact, you'll also look more trim and compact.

7

Getting Started

Now, let's stop talking about metabolism and start doing something about it. If you're like my patients, you probably can't wait to begin. What are we waiting for? Let's go!

How Much Should You Lose?

The first step is to work out how many pounds you need to lose. You may already be well aware of how overweight you are. Just as a check, I'm providing you with the following height/weight charts so you can determine your ideal weight. These heights are without shoes, and the weights without clothing. Separate charts are provided for women and men.

These charts are based on the most up-to-date calculations from worldwide weight control experts.

Based on your height, find your desired weight on the chart. The chart gives you an average desirable weight and a range of acceptable weights. If you are a woman and are five feet six inches tall, your desirable weight would be 128 pounds. Your weight would still be in a *healthy* range if it was between 114 and 146 pounds. This range allows you to take into account your body frame and personal preference. The five-feet-six-inch-tall woman may be able to maintain and regulate her weight better at 135 pounds than 128 pounds. Another five-feet-six-inch-tall woman may still feel fat at 135 pounds. Her clothes may fit better, and she may feel more attractive at 120 pounds.

Desired Weight Chart
(in pounds)
Women

Height	Average Acceptable Weight	Acceptable Weight Range
4'10"	102	92-119
4'11"	104	94-122
5'0"	107	96-125
5'1"	110	99-128
5'2"	113	102-131
5'3"	116	105-134
5'4"	120	108-138
5'5"	123	111-142
5'6"	128	114-146
5'7"	132	118-150
5'8"	136	122-154
5'9"	140	126-158
5'10"	144	130-163
5'11"	148	134-168
6'0"	152	138-173

Men

Height	Average Acceptable Weight	Acceptable Weight Range
5'2"	123	112-141
5'3"	127	115-144
5'4"	130	118-148
5'5"	133	121-152
5'6"	136	124-156
5'7"	140	128-161
5'8"	145	132-166
5'9"	149	136-170
5'10"	153	140-174
5'11"	158	144-179
6'0"	162	148-184
6'1"	166	152-189
6'2"	171	156-194
6'3"	176	160-199
6'4"	181	164-204

Choose a weight that is right for you. Just make sure it falls within the healthy range on the chart. And you don't get any extra pounds for age either. Older people should be just as slim as younger ones.

How Often Should You Weigh Yourself?

Before you get started, weigh yourself on a good bathroom or physician's scales. If you have old scales that never seem to be accurate, throw them out and get new ones. Tape a piece of paper on the inside of your bathroom door, and every time you weigh, write down the date and your weight.

Here are my rules about weighing:

1. Weigh yourself on the first morning you begin the diet.
2. After the first weigh-in, weigh yourself once a week and once a week *only*.
3. Always weigh yourself first thing in the morning (before breakfast) and on the same day each week.
4. Always weigh without clothing or while wearing light underclothes.

You *must* resist the urge to weigh every day during the diet. Those of you who are addicted to the scales must avoid weighing several times a day! If you're like most overweight people, you have two extremes. If you're fat and not dieting, you'll avoid scales (and perhaps mirrors) like the plague. If you're dieting, you'll weigh yourself almost every hour to see if you're losing weight. Neither of these patterns is good for you.

Normal daily fluctuations in weight and temporary plateaux will discourage you if you weigh too often. Besides, the scales only measure your total body weight. They don't tell you a thing about your fat content, muscle content, or metabolism.

Hide your scales if you have to, but *weigh only once a week*.

What Other Measures Should You Take?

Because you'll be losing body fat *and* firming up your lean body tissue, the scale won't tell you the whole story of your progress. The Hilton Head Metabolism Diet will not only make you lighter, but also a lot slimmer – and there's quite a difference. When you lose fifteen pounds on the Hilton Head Metabolism Diet, you'll look like you've lost twenty. I'm giving you an extra five pounds of weight loss absolutely free. One of my patients put it this way: 'I lost fifteen pounds and my friends couldn't get over the difference. Everyone said I looked like a new person, fifteen years younger. I've never had that happen when I've lost weight before.'

To find out how much slimmer you're becoming, you need to take your body measurements. As you'll remember from Chapter 3, you can keep track of how much actual fat you're losing just by knowing your waist and thigh measurements.

The following body measurements should be taken with a tape measure *once every two weeks:*

1. Chest – measure around your chest at the nipple line.
2. Abdomen – measure around your waist at the level of your belly button (at the top of your pelvis).
3. Hips – measure around your hips at about midbuttock level.
4. Upper thigh – measure around the uppermost part of your thighs completely around your body.
5. Mid thigh – measure around your right thigh halfway between your knee and the uppermost part of your leg.

6. Upper arm – measure halfway between your shoulder and elbow, with your arm hanging down naturally.

Make sure you keep a written record of these measurements each time you take them.

Check with Your Doctor

Before you begin this or any diet, consult your doctor. If you have particular medical or dietary problems, he will need to supervise your progress closely.

The Hilton Head Metabolism Diet plan is a healthy nutritional and exercise programme that has been approved by physicians. In fact, some of my most successful and enthusiastic patients have been medical doctors.

8

The Hilton Head Metabolism Diet

Now you're ready to begin. Remember, you're not just going to lose weight. Also, and more importantly, you'll be changing your metabolism. After following the Hilton Head Metabolism Diet you'll finally be able to eat normally without having to think about dieting ever again!

Right from the start of the diet, you will also notice two things that may surprise you:

1. You *will not* be hungry.
2. You *will* have loads of energy.

Many people are sure they will feel hungry, deprived, and fatigued on a diet. However, the Hilton Head Metabolism Diet is so well balanced and has such positive effects on your metabolism that you'll feel energetic and completely satisfied. After two weeks on the diet, a busy housewife said to me, 'I have so much energy I can't believe it. I'm able to get twice as much work done, and have energy to spare. I'm finally finding time to do things for me – to do the things I really enjoy. And I'm a lot less irritable with the family, too. I haven't felt hungry once since I started the Metabolism Diet, even though I'm eating so much less than I usually do!'

Phases of the Hilton Head Metabolism Diet

The Hilton Head Metabolism Diet is different from any other diet you've ever been on. Because I am trying to help you change your metabolism, you *must* follow my diet exactly as it is prescribed. Do not make any changes for any reason. If you do, then the plan won't do what it's designed to do. You might lose weight, but you'll still have to fight to keep it off, because you did *not* change your metabolism. I want this to be your very last diet, so follow my instructions to the letter.

As mentioned in Chaper 4, the Hilton Head Metabolism Diet has three phases. *You must go through all three phases to be successful.* They are as follows:

1. LOW-CAL Phase
   Always begin with the Low-cal menu plan. This phase is designed for maximum weight loss. Follow these menus for *two weeks*.

2. BOOSTER Phase
   After two weeks, switch to the Booster menu plan for *one week*. This phase allows about 300 more calories each day and is designed to boost your metabolic rate. You *must* switch to this Booster Phase for one week after two weeks in the Low-cal phase.

3. REENTRY Phase
   When you get within one to three pounds of your goal weight, switch to the Reentry menu plan. This phase enables your metabolism to increase gradually, getting it ready for maintenance. If you skip this phase, you run the risk of gaining some of your weight back within the first two weeks after the diet is over.

To make these phases as easy as possible, I am providing you with weekly charts to follow, based on how much weight you have to lose. These charts will tell you which menu plan to follow during each week of the diet. They are based on the most typical weight loss patterns of my patients.

Separate listings are given for men and for women, because men lose weight (because of metabolism) at a faster rate than women. Please note that women wanting to lose ten pounds and men wanting to lose either ten or fifteen pounds only, need to follow the Low-cal menu phase for one week before switching to the Booster Phase. All others follow a two-week Low-cal, then a one-week Booster sequence.

Since people lose weight at varying rates, you may have to adjust these sequences slightly. For example, let's suppose you have twenty pounds to lose. After three weeks of dieting you have lost eighteen pounds. You are now ready for the Reentry Phase. Even though the chart says you should follow the Low-cal menus during Week 4, ignore this and go directly to the Reentry menus. Whenever you are within one to three pounds of your goal, switch to Reentry no matter what the chart says.

Let's suppose that the reverse situation happens. You have twenty pounds to lose, but after four weeks you've lost only sixteen pounds. The chart says you should go to Reentry during Week 5. However, you haven't progressed far enough with your weight loss. Ignore the chart and stay on the Low-cal menus for one more week before going to Reentry.

The sequence is really quite simple, and most people can follow the charts. As a general rule, however, just follow the weekly sequence of Low-cal, Low-cal, Booster, Low-cal, Low-cal, Booster until you get within one to three pounds of your goal. When you get to this level, whenever it occurs, switch to Reentry. After one week on Reentry you should be ready for maintenance. You will have made it!

Sequence of Menu Plans

10-lb Plan		
Week	*WOMEN*	*MEN*
1	Low-cal	Low-cal
2	Booster	Reentry
3	Reentry	—

15-lb Plan		
Week	*WOMEN*	*MEN*
1	Low-cal	Low-cal
2	Low-cal	Booster
3	Booster	Reentry
4	Reentry	—

20-lb Plan		
Week	*WOMEN*	*MEN*
1	Low-cal	Low-cal
2	Low-cal	Low-cal
3	Booster	Booster
4	Low-cal	Reentry
5	Reentry	—

25-lb Plan		
Week	*WOMEN*	*MEN*
1	Low-cal	Low-cal
2	Low-cal	Low-cal
3	Booster	Booster
4	Low-cal	Low-cal
5	Low-cal	Reentry
6	Reentry	—

30-lb Plan		
Week	*WOMEN*	*MEN*
1	Low-cal	Low-cal
2	Low-cal	Low-cal
3	Booster	Booster
4	Low-cal	Low-cal
5	Low-cal	Low-cal
6	Booster	Reentry
7	Reentry	—

40-lb Plan		
Week	*WOMEN*	*MEN*
1	Low-cal	Low-cal
2	Low-cal	Low-cal
3	Booster	Booster
4	Low-cal	Low-cal
5	Low-cal	Low-cal
6	Booster	Booster
7	Low-cal	Low-cal
8	Low-cal	Reentry
9	Reentry	—

50-lb Plan		
Week	*WOMEN*	*MEN*
1	Low-cal	Low-cal
2	Low-cal	Low-cal
3	Booster	Booster
4	Low-cal	Low-cal
5	Low-cal	Low-cal
6	Booster	Booster
7	Low-cal	Low-cal
8	Low-cal	Low-cal
9	Booster	Booster
10	Low-cal	Reentry
11	Reentry	—

If you have more than fifty pounds to lose, keep alternating two weeks of Low-cal with one week of Booster until you're ready for Reentry.

The Metabo-Meal

The Hilton Head Metabolism Diet gives you *four* delicious meals every day. You *must* eat all four meals for the diet to work properly. *Never ever skip a meal under any circumstances.*

In addition to breakfast, lunch, and dinner, you will be eating what I call the *metabo-meal*. This fourth meal helps to stimulate your metabolism through the thermic effect. The metabo-meal may be eaten in the evening *or* in the mid- to late afternoon. If you generally eat dinner between five o'clock and seven o'clock, I recommend you eat the metabo-meal in the late evening, between 9:00

P.M. and 10:30 P.M. If you eat dinner later than 7:00 P.M., you might prefer to eat your metabo-meal in the afternoon, between 3:30 P.M. and 5:00 P.M. Try to keep about the same time interval between your four meals.

Basic Rules of the Hilton Head Metabolism Diet

1. Eat everything exactly as it is prescribed. Avoid substitutions unless specified. If you are allergic to certain foods or if they aren't available, substitution lists are provided in Chaper 19.
2. Don't eat anything more than the meals assigned.
3. *Never skip a meal*.
4. Drink plenty of fluids – water, low-calorie drinks, iced tea. Coffee and hot tea are allowed, but make sure you drink at least two to three glasses of water per day. Avoid caloric drinks such as fruit juices, or liquids that are high in sodium, such as tomato juice and beef extract.
5. Do *not* add table salt to your food. It's simply not healthy and may result in water retention, which will mask your weekly weight losses. You get plenty of sodium (salt) naturally in the foods on the diet.
6. Remove all visible fat from meat, and remove the skin from chicken before eating it.
7. Avoid *all* alcoholic beverages. No beer, wine, or spirits until you lose your weight.
8. Buy only *fresh* fruits and vegetables. If these are not available, buy frozen. *Never* use tinned fruits or vegetables.

Now let's get started. Here are the Low-cal menus. Keep

in mind that the number of ounces indicated for fish, meat, or chicken refers to *cooked* ounces. You should buy about two ounces more than you need to allow for shrinkage during cooking.

Low-Cal menus

BREAKFAST EVERY DAY

Cereal 25g (1oz) – Choose cereals that are low in sugar content, such as Special K, 40% Bran, Shredded Wheat, Wheaties, Raisin Bran, oatmeal, or Puffed Wheat.

Milk 100ml (4fl oz) – Low-fat (2%) or skimmed milk only.

Fruit (½ piece) – Choice of orange, banana, pear, apple, grapefruit, or peach.

Coffee or tea – Sugar substitute and/or dash of low-fat or skimmed milk may be added if desired.

MONDAY

BREAKFAST:

Low-cal breakfast

LUNCH:

Fruit Platter:
    Strawberries 60g (2½oz)
    Honeydew melon 25g (1oz) (Substitute fruit in season.)
    Cantaloupe 25g (1oz)
    Cottage cheese 50g (2oz)
    Lettuce (a few leaves under the fruit)

DINNER:

Baked chicken (150g (5oz) or 2 breasts)
Baked potato (1 medium, no butter)
Vegetable: choice of green beans, broccoli, asparagus
    100g (4oz)
Strawberries 60g (2½oz)
Natural yoghurt (1 tablespoon over fruit)

METABO-MEAL:

Cinnamon toast (2 slices of thin-sliced wholemeal bread
sprinkled lightly with cinnamon or mixture of cinnamon
and artificial sweetener and toasted under the grill)

TUESDAY

BREAKFAST:

Low-cal breakfast

LUNCH:

Egg (1 whole egg, any way. If fried, brush pan *lightly* with
    oil)
Wholemeal bread (1 slice, toasted)
Grapefruit (½)

DINNER:

Baked or grilled fish (175g (6oz) of any type, no butter)
Rice (white or brown, 75g (3oz))
Vegetables: choice of two – broccoli, carrots, green beans,
    cauliflower, asparagus, spinach (100g (4oz) each)
Orange slices (50g (2oz) with dash of natural yoghurt if
    desired)

METABO-MEAL:

Smalled tossed salad (2 tablespoons diet dressing)
Apple (½)

WEDNESDAY

BREAKFAST:

Low-cal breakfast

LUNCH:

Tuna fish (75g (3oz) water-packed)
Lettuce (¼ small head)
Tomato (½ medium)
Cucumber slices (10 slices)
Diet salad dressing (2 tablespoons)

DINNER:

Grilled, lean hamburger 175g (6oz)
Egg noodles 50g (2oz)
Vegetable: choice of green beans, broccoli, asparagus
   100g (4oz)

METABO-MEAL:

Cereal (15g (½oz); choice of Shredded Wheat or 40% Bran)
Milk (100ml (4fl oz) low-fat or skimmed)
Banana (½)

THURSDAY

BREAKFAST:

Low-cal breakfast

LUNCH:

Tossed salad (large salad bowl with lettuce, tomato, cucumber, radish mix; 2 tablespoons diet dressing)
Roll (1 small hard roll; 1 tablespoon diet margarine)

DINNER:

Baked chicken (150g (5oz) or 2 breasts)
New potatoes (2 or 3 small)
Vegetable: choice of spinach, green beans, broccoli 100g (4oz)
Fruit: choice of cantaloupe (⅛) or strawberries/blackberries 60g (2½oz)

METABO-MEAL:

Cottage cheese 50g (2oz)
Apple (½)

FRIDAY

BREAKFAST:

Low-cal breakfast

LUNCH:

Whole tomato stuffed with chicken salad (75g (3oz) – see recipe in Chapter 20)

DINNER:

Grilled fish or prawns (175–225g (6–8oz) of any type)
Corn on the cob (1 medium)
Small tossed salad (with 2 tablespoons diet dressing)
Peach (1 whole, sliced and topped with 25g (1oz) natural yoghurt) (Substitute fruit in season.)

METABO-MEAL:

Raw vegetable platter (mixture of 6 each of raw carrot sticks, celery, radishes, and cauliflower with diet dip, if desired. See recipe for dip in Chapter 20.)

SATURDAY

BREAKFAST:

Low-cal breakfast

LUNCH:

Fruit salad:
    Cottage cheese 50g (2oz)
    Lettuce (¼ head)
    Orange (½)
    Apple (½)
    Grapes 75g (3oz)

DINNER:

Grilled steak (125–150g (4–5oz) of any type, all visible fat removed)

Baked potato (1 medium, with 2 tablespoons diet margarine)

Vegetable: choice of courgettes, broccoli, asparagus 100g (4oz)

METABO-MEAL:

Sliced banana (1 whole, lightly sprinkled with cinnamon-artificial sweetener mixture and toasted under grill)

SUNDAY

BREAKFAST:

Low-cal breakfast

LUNCH:

Omelette:
  Egg whites (whites of 3 eggs)
  Cottage cheese 50g (2oz)
  Onion (⅛ small)
  Green pepper (25g (1oz) chopped)
  Mushrooms (25g (1oz) chopped)
Note: Fry egg whites lightly in frying or omelette pan, brushing lightly with oil. As egg whites set, add cottage cheese, onion, green pepper, and mushrooms, and fold over omelette to cover filling.
Apple (½)

DINNER:

Spaghetti (50g (2oz) cooked)
Meatless sauce (100g (4oz) commercially prepared sauce, or use recipe in Chapter 20)
Parmesan cheese (sprinkled lightly over spaghetti)
Tossed salad (small bowl of lettuce, tomato, cucumber, radish mix, with 2 tablespoons diet dressing)
Roll or bread (1 small hard roll or 2 medium slices of French bread, with *no* butter)

METABO-MEAL:

Fruit platter:
  Apple (½)
  Banana (½)
  Raisins (1 tablespoon)
Note: Slice and mix fruit together.

Second Week of the Low-cal Phase

During the second week of the Low-cal Phase, simply repeat the menus from the first week. Then, as I have instructed, switch over to the Booster menus listed in Chapter 9.

Substitutions and Variations

Although I have instructed you to stick strictly to these menus, I realize that substitutions and variations are sometimes necessary. Generally, these changes are only needed when

1. You are unable to buy fruits or vegetables because they are not in season.
2. You have a lot of weight to lose and, because of the length of the diet for you, more variation is necessary.
3. You are allergic to specific foods such as fish, milk products, or certain fruit.

In Chapters 19 and 20 I have provided detailed substitution and variation lists for fruits, vegetables, potatoes, and main courses. For example, I give you my secrets for five separate ways to prepare low calorie potato dishes. In addition, I've included a variety of recipes for you dietary gourmets who want to experiment a bit. Do *not* make any substitutions of your own. You may, without realizing it, change the nutritional balance of the diet. As I stated earlier, the proportions of protein, carbohydrates, and fats on the diet are *extremely* important. When making any necessary adjustments, you must always substitute a

protein for a protein and a carbohydrate for a carbohydrate. Refer to my substitution lists before making any
changes.

Generally speaking, the. fewer substitutes the better.
People who follow the menus strictly as given have the
most success.

Easy-to-Follow Menus

In looking over the Low-cal menus, you've probably no-
ticed how practical and easy-to-follow they are. The meals
consist of common, everyday foods that are easy to buy.
No fancy or expensive 'diet' foods are included. Plenty of
variation in day-to-day meals is provided. You'll be
especially thankful for this variety if you've ever been on a
diet that allows only one type of food, such as grapefruit,
day after day.

One of my patients told me: 'Your diet is so easy. It
takes very little time to prepare, and I can serve my family
the same kind of food – just more of it. I don't have to
prepare two separate sets of meals for myself and the
family as I had to do on other diets. And, even when we
occasionally eat out, I can order exactly what's on my
Low-cal menu. Thank goodness for the Hilton Head
Metabolism Diet.'

9
The Booster Phase

After two weeks on the Low-cal menus, you must switch to the Booster menus *for one week*. The Booster Phase gives you about 1100 calories per day – 300 more than the Low-cal Phase. Do *not* hesitate to switch to the Booster menus. Remember, fewer calories are not necessarily better than more calories. That's an old attitude of yours that must be changed.

Patients say to me, 'If I'm losing weight on 800 calories, why eat more? In fact, maybe I'd lose more if I ate even fewer calories.' *Wrong. Wrong. Wrong.* This is just the kind of thinking that caused your metabolism problem in the first place.

You *must* enter the slightly higher calorie Booster Phase for one week for my system to work. We have to keep jolting your metabolism. Prolonged dieting with low calories puts it to sleep. That's just what we're trying to prevent.

And you *will* lose weight during the Booster Phase. You'll continue to lose because, even though you're eating slightly more, you are also burning more. Your metabolism has speeded up. In fact, most people lose just as much during the Booster weeks as they do during the Low-cal weeks.

Keep in mind that this is a carefully worked out system that has been tested on many, many patients. It definitely works. But, it only works if you follow the system *exactly* as it has been developed for you. Forget about your relatives and friends and do *not* listen to advice from them. I am giving you the *only* way to achieve permanent weight control. You must be as zealous as a new religious convert. Follow me to a slim life for ever. Just make sure you follow me step by step, making no changes on your own.

An End to Dieting Monotony

In addition to its metabolic effects, the Booster Phase eliminates the boredom and monotony characteristic of other diets. Most dieters simply get tired of the same old routine, the same old food. They begin to feel rebellious. Monotony is indeed the dieter's enemy.

The Booster menus provide a refreshing change of pace. After every two weeks of the Low-cal menus, you are allowed not only more to eat, but a different variety of food – bagels, cream cheese, muffins, lamb, veal, roast beef, grilled cheese sandwiches, and even popcorn. You'll still be dieting, but it won't seem like it. You'll always have the Booster weeks to look forward to. This is particularly important if you have a lot of weight to lose.

A patient of mine who lost fifty-two pounds put it this way: 'I *never* felt bored with the Hilton Head Metabolism Diet. The variety was so plentiful, especially during the Booster weeks, I almost forgot I was dieting. On other diets I used to get bored with the same foods over and over again. I never lasted more than a few days. I felt so deprived. Now I've lost fifty-two pounds, boosted my metabolism, and never once felt sorry for myself.'

What Calories Have Been Added?

In keeping with the nutritional influences on metabolism that I discussed in Chapter 4, most of the added calories during the Booster Phase are carbohydrates. Remember that carbohydrates – fruits, vegetables, potatoes, bread, pasta – are good for you and good for your metabolism. I have added more bread, vegetables, and fruit. You'll also notice that more diet margarine, diet salad dressings, and even mayonnaise are allowed during the Booster weeks. A little more fat is actually good for you during this time. Even so, you'll still be eating a low-fat diet.

I've added more variety and switched fish and chicken days around a bit. Most of the extra calories have been added to the lunches and metabo-meals. Most people are satisfied with 150 to 200 calories at breakfast, and my dinner menus even during the Low-cal weeks are plentiful. In fact, at the beginning of the diet some people even complain they can't eat all the dinner. It is important to eat *all* the food at every meal.

When to Begin and End the Booster Phase

As a general rule, follow the Sequence of Menu Plans on pages 61 to 63 in Chapter 8. That will tell you when to begin and end both the Low-cal and Booster phases, based on the amount of weight you have to lose. Unless you only have about ten pounds to lose, you'll begin to eat the Booster menus after every two weeks of Low-cal. Always stay on the Booster menus for one full week. Then switch back to Low-cal for two weeks. Keep switching back and forth until you lose your excess weight.

Continue to follow the basic rules for the Hilton Head Metabolism Diet (see pages 64 to 65 in Chapter 8). And remember, never skip any meal – eat four meals a day, every day.

Booster menus

BREAKFAST EVERY DAY

Cereal 25g (1oz) – Choose cereals that are low in sugar content, such as Special K, 40% Bran, Shredded Wheat, Wheaties, Raisin Bran, oatmeal, or Puffed Wheat.

Milk 100ml (4fl oz) – Low-fat (2%) or skimmed milk only.

Fruit (1 whole) – Choice of orange, banana, pear, apple, grapefruit, or peach.

Coffee or tea – Sugar substitute and/or dash of low-fat or skimmed milk may be added if desired.

MONDAY

BREAKFAST:

Booster breakfast

LUNCH:

Tuna fish sandwich:
   Wholemeal bread (2 slices)
   Tuna (50g (2oz) water-packed tinned tuna, mixed with
     1 teaspoon mayonnaise)
   Lettuce
Peach (½ small)

DINNER:

Poussin (approximately 150g (5oz) of meat)
New potatoes (2–3 small)
Vegetable: choice of carrots, green beans, broccoli,
   asparagus 100g (4oz)

Strawberries or blackberries (60g (2½oz), topped with a tablespoon natural yoghurt)

METABO-MEAL:

Muffin (1 whole, toasted and topped with 1 tablespoon diet margarine)

TUESDAY

BREAKFAST:

Booster breakfast

LUNCH:

Chicken salad (75g (3oz) chicken with 1 teaspoon mayonnaise and 1 teaspoon chopped celery)
Lettuce (a few leaves under chicken salad)
Tomato (½, sliced)

DINNER:

Baked or grilled fish (175g (6oz) of any type, *no* butter)
Baked potato (1 medium, no butter)
Vegetables: choice of two – broccoli, carrots, green beans, cauliflower, asparagus, spinach (100g (4oz) each)
Apple-raisin mix (½ apple, diced, mixed with 1 tablespoon raisins)

METABO-MEAL:

Popcorn (100g (4oz) of popped popcorn with 1 tablespoon diet margarine, *no* salt)

WEDNESDAY

BREAKFAST:

Booster breakfast

LUNCH:

Cottage cheese 75g (3oz)
Cantaloupe (¼, cut in wedges)
Strawberries (60g (2½oz), sliced)
Lettuce (a few leaves under fruit and cottage cheese)

DINNER:

Roast lamb or veal (150g (5oz), all visible fat removed)
Baked potato (1 medium with 1 teaspoon diet margarine)
Vegetable: choice of green beans, broccoli, asparagus
    100g (4oz)

METABO-MEAL:

Raw vegetable platter (mixture of raw carrot sticks,
    celery, cauliflower, radishes)
Cream crackers (6, unsalted)

THURSDAY

BREAKFAST:

Booster breakfast

LUNCH:

Eggs (2 any way. If fried, brush pan lightly with oil)
Wholemeal bread, (1 slice, toasted)
Grapefruit (½)

DINNER:

Spaghetti (100g (4oz) cooked)

Meatless sauce (150g (5oz) commercially prepared sauce, or use recipe in Chapter 20)

Parmesan cheese (sprinkled lightly over spaghetti)

Bread (2 medium slices of French bread, with 1 tablespoon diet margarine)

METABO-MEAL:

Fruit: choice of two – banana, orange, pear, apple, grapefruit, peach

FRIDAY

BREAKFAST:

Booster breakfast

LUNCH:

Tossed salad (large salad bowl with lettuce, tomato, cucumber, radish, pepper, and carrot, mixed together with 3 tablespoons diet dressing)

Fruit: choice of apple or pear

DINNER:

Grilled fish or prawns (175–225g (6–8oz) any type with fish or prawn sauce – see recipe in Chapter 20)

Rice (white or brown, cooked, 175g (6oz))

Vegetables: choice of two – broccoli, carrots, green beans, cauliflower, asparagus, spinach (100g (4oz) each)

Orange slices (50g (2oz), with 1 tablespoon natural or lemon yoghurt)

METABO-MEAL:

Bagel (1 whole with ½ tablespoon cream cheese)

SATURDAY

BREAKFAST:

Booster breakfast

LUNCH:

Open grilled cheese and tomato sandwich (2 slices of white or wholemeal bread, each topped with slices of tomato and low-fat cheese (e.g. Edam) and grilled lightly)

DINNER:

Roast beef 150g (5oz)
Baked potato (1 medium, no butter)
Vegetable: choice of courgettes, broccoli, asparagus 100g (4oz)
Tossed salad (small bowl of lettuce, onions, tomato, cucumbers, and radishes, mixed with 2 tablespoons diet dressing)

METABO-MEAL:

Cereal: choice of Shredded Wheat or 40% Bran 15g (½oz)
Milk (100ml (4 fl oz) low-fat or skimmed)
Banana (1 whole)

SUNDAY

BREAKFAST:

Booster breakfast

LUNCH:

Egg salad sandwich:
   Rye or wholemeal bread (2 slices)
   Egg salad (1 whole egg, hard-boiled, chopped, with 1
      tablespoon mayonnaise)
   Lettuce
Strawberries (60g (2½oz) – substitute fruit in season)

DINNER:

Turkey or chicken 150g (5oz)
Rice (white or brown, cooked 75g (3oz))
Vegetables: choice of two – spinach, green beans,
   broccoli, carrots, asparagus, cauliflower (100g (4oz)
   each)
Fruit: choice of orange, apple, peach, pear (½)

METABO-MEAL:

Repeat your favourite metabo-meal from the Booster
menus.

10

The Reentry Phase

As you continue with the Low-cal and Booster phases, you should weigh yourself every Monday morning, keeping careful track of your weight. On the Monday that you are within two pounds or less of your goal, you are ready for the Reentry Phase.

The case of George, a forty-three-year-old lawyer patient of mine, illustrates the proper timing of this phase. Over the past ten years George had gradually put on more and more weight until he weighed 200 pounds. He felt fat, unattractive, old, and lethargic. At six feet one inch, his ideal weight fell within the range of 152 to 189. He looked and felt his best at 175 pounds. When he discovered the Hilton Head Metabolism Diet, he was elated. He wanted to lose his fat image and be able to maintain a slim body for the rest of his life.

He began the diet on 19 November 1981, determined to trim down *permanently*. His weekly weight losses and the timing sequence of phases he went through are presented below.

Weeks	Weight	Total Loss	Phase
Prior to diet	200 lb	—	—
Week 1	190 lb	10 lb	Low-cal
Week 2	184 lb	16 lb	Low-cal
Week 3	180 lb	20 lb	Booster
Week 4	176 lb	24 lb	Low-cal
Week 5	174 lb	26 lb	Reentry

When he stood on his scale after four weeks, he weighed 176 pounds, only one pound from his goal. He was ready for the Reentry Phase. He was close enough to his goal to get his metabolism ready for normal eating again. If he went directly from the Low-cal Phase to normal maintenance eating, he would probably gain two to three pounds of his weight back again. As is the universal case, his metabolism would still be somewhat lowered from dieting. He would be eating a maintenance number of calories (e.g. 2800 per day) but gaining rather than maintaining, because his thermostat hadn't been turned back up yet. In addition, water weight is often gained when going too quickly from a diet to a higher number of calories. This is quite normal and is usually no more than one or two pounds. The Reentry Phase counteracts both of these negative side effects of dieting.

By switching to the Reentry menus, consisting of approximately 1500 calories per day (about halfway between Low-cal and maintenance), George eased his metabolism up to where it belonged: he lost two more pounds during Reentry. After the Reentry week was over, both he and his metabolism were ready for normal eating again. Only this time George weighed a slim 174 pounds and could eat as much as he did before, without gaining weight. George still keeps in touch with me and is doing just fine. He maintains a weight between 174 and 176 and continues with the Metabolism Maintenance Plan.

The Reentry Meals

As the calories increase from 800 in the Low-cal Phase to 1100 in the Booster Phase to 1500 in the Reentry Phase, you'll be getting not only more food, but more choices.

The main nutrients added in the Reentry Phase are carbohydrates, with some fat and some protein. Remember, your eventual nutritional balance at maintenance should consist of 15 to 20 per cent protein, 50 to 55 per cent carbohydrates, and 25 to 30 per cent fat.

When eating the Reentry meals, you'll notice more bread, pasta, and vegetables. I have added higher calorie vegetables such as corn, peas, and broad beans for variety. You'll also notice that I'm getting you back to nondietetic products such as regular salad dressing, mayonnaise, and cheese. More sandwiches are included. Also I'm now allowing fruit juice for breakfast. At the lower number of allowed calories, fruit juices were not worth the added input. You were better off with fresh fruit. Now there's more flexibility.

I've also added more fibre foods in the form of wholemeal bread and bran cereals. High fibre foods are healthy for you and help with elimination problems. They also speed up the passage of food and waste through the digestive tract so that less of it is absorbed into your system. The less absorbed, the fewer calories you take in. Unfortunately, some high fibre foods such as whole-grain bread, cereal, and bran biscuits are relatively high in calories. That's why I've had to add them gradually. Once you're off the diet, however, they should be a regular part of your menu plan. I'll have more to say about this later.

Now for the Reentry menus. Keep following the dietary rules set out in Chapter 8. Stay on the Reentry menus for one week. If you still have not quite reached your goal at that time (for example, if you're still one pound away), you may stay with the Reentry menus for one more week if you wish. People who have a lot of weight to lose and who must stay on the diet for quite a while will need to spend two weeks in the Reentry Phase. Their metabolism must make a big adjustment and therefore they should be phased into normal eating more gradually.

Reentry Menus

BREAKFAST EVERY DAY

Fruit juice (100 ml (4 fl oz)) – Choice of unsweetened or fresh grapefruit, orange, apricot, or prune juice.

Cereal (25g (1 oz)) – Choice of 40% Bran, All-Bran, Raisin Bran, or other high fibre cereal.

Milk (100 ml (4 fl oz)) – Low-fat (2%) or skimmed milk only.

Fruit (1 whole) – Choice of orange, banana, pear, apple, grapefruit, peach, melon.

MONDAY

BREAKFAST:

Reentry breakfast

LUNCH:

Chicken salad sandwich:
  Chicken salad (75g (3oz) diced chicken mixed with 1 tablespoon mayonnaise)
  Wholemeal bread (2 pieces, thin-sliced)
  Lettuce (1 or 2 leaves on sandwich)
Pear (½)

DINNER:

Baked or grilled fish, prawns, crab, or lobster meat (175g (6oz), *no* butter)

Tossed salad (small bowl of lettuce, tomato, cucumber, onion, radish mixture with 2 tablespoons *non*dietetic salad dressing)

Sweet potato (1 whole, with ½ tablespoon diet margarine)

Vegetable: choice of carrots, green beans, broccoli, asparagus, spinach 100g (4oz)

Strawberries (60g (2½oz), topped with 1 tablespoon natural or lemon yoghurt)

METABO-MEAL:

Muffin (1 whole, with 1 tablespoon margarine *or* 1 tablespoon *non*dietetic jam or jelly)

Grapes 100g (4oz)

TUESDAY

BREAKFAST:

Reentry breakfast

LUNCH:

Hamburger:

   Hamburger roll (1 whole)

   Beef patty (75g (3oz) grilled lean beef, topped with ½ tablespoon mayonnaise *or* 2 tablespoons ketchup)

   Lettuce (1 or 2 leaves)

   Tomato (1 slice)

DINNER:

Macaroni and cheese 100g (4oz)

Asparagus spears (4)

Tomato (1 whole, grilled and topped with tarragon or dill)

METABO-MEAL:

Cream crackers (6)
Milk (1 cup low-fat or skimmed)

WEDNESDAY

BREAKFAST:

Reentry breakfast

LUNCH:

Cottage cheese 75g (3oz)
Cantaloupe (½, cut in wedges)
Strawberries (60g (2½oz), Sliced)
Lettuce (2 or 3 leaves)
Roll (1 medium, any type, with 1 tablespoon diet margarine)

DINNER:

Steak (50g (5oz) any type, grilled, with all visible fat removed)
Baked potato (1 whole, with 1 tablespoon diet margarine)
Vegetable: choice of corn, peas, broad beans 100g (4oz)
Spinach salad (small bowl of raw spinach, onions, radishes, cucumber, and carrots with 2 tablespoons diet salad dressing)

METABO-MEAL:

Bagel (1 whole, with 2 tablespoons cream cheese)
Fruit: choice of orange, apple, pear (1 whole)

THURSDAY

BREAKFAST:

Reentry breakfast

LUNCH:

Omelette (2-egg omelette filled with tomatoes, peppers, onions, and cheddar cheese)
Bread or roll (2 pieces, with 2 tablespoons diet margarine)

DINNER:

Baked chicken (150g (5oz) or 2 breasts)
New potatoes (2 to 3 small)
Vegetable: choice of carrots, asparagus, spinach, courgettes, green beans 225g (8oz)
Baked apple (1 whole, cut in half and topped with cinnamon and brown sugar substitute, baked for 20 to 30 minutes at 180°C (350°F), Gas 4)

METABO-MEAL:

Raw vegetable platter (mixture of 6 each of raw carrot sticks, celery, radishes, and cauliflower)
Melba toast or Ryvita (4 pieces, with 2 tablespoons diet margarine)
Juice: choice of orange, apple, grapefruit, prune, apricot 100ml (4 fl oz)

FRIDAY

BREAKFAST:

Reentry breakfast

LUNCH:

Tuna fish sandwich:
    Tuna (50g (2oz), with 1 tablespoon mayonnaise)
    Bran bread (2 slices)
    Lettuce (1 or 2 leaves)
    Tomato (2 slices)
Peach (1 whole)

DINNER:

Baked or grilled fish (175g (6 oz), any type)
Rice (white or brown, cooked 175g (6oz), topped with 1
    tablespoon diet margarine)
Vegetable: choice of corn, peas, broad beans 225g (8oz)
Orange slices 100g (4oz)

METABO-MEAL:

Yoghurt (225ml (8 fl oz) of any fruit-flavoured yoghurt)

SATURDAY

BREAKFAST:

Reentry breakfast

LUNCH:

Large salad (large salad bowl with lettuce, tomato,
    onions, carrots, pepper, radishes, 50g (2oz) diced
    chicken or turkey, and croutons, topped with 2
    tablespoons *non*dietetic salad dressing)

DINNER:

Roast beef, lamb, or veal (150g (5oz), all visible fat re-
moved)
Baked potato (1 whole, with 2 tablespoons sour cream)
Vegetable: choice of asparagus, green beans, beetroot,
carrots, broccoli, spinach 225g (8oz)
Bread or roll (2 pieces, *no* butter or margarine)

METABO-MEAL:

Popcorn (100g (4oz) of popped corn with 1 tablespoon
diet margarine – *no* salt)
Fruit: choice of apple, orange, pear, peach, melon
(1 whole)

SUNDAY

BREAKFAST:

Reentry breakfast

LUNCH:

Open grilled cheese and tomato sandwich (2 slices of
wholemeal or rye bread each topped with slices of
tomato and low-fat cheese, e.g. Edam, grilled lightly
Fruit: choice of apple, orange, pear (½)

DINNER:

Spaghetti (225g (8oz) cooked)
Meatless sauce (175g (6oz) commercially prepared sauce,
or use recipe in Chapter 20)

Parmesan cheese (sprinkled lightly over spaghetti)
Bread (2 medium slices of French bread with 1 tablespoon
   diet margarine)

METABO-MEAL:

Repeat your favourite metabo-meal from the Reentry
menus.

11

Questions and Answers about the Hilton Head Metabolism Diet

Q. *Will I need to take vitamins on the Hilton Head Metabolism Diet?*

A. While you are in the Low-cal and Booster phases, I recommend you take a multivitamin with a mineral supplement. Any name brand or generic multivitamin will do. You do not need any special vitamin supplements. If you stick to my maintenance plan after the diet is over, you won't need any vitamins.

Q. *How much fluid should I drink on the Hilton Head Metabolism Diet?*

A. Because you'll be eating less salt and exercising more than you're used to, I suggest you drink plenty of fluid. You should drink at least three to four glasses of water, iced tea, or low-calorie drinks each day.

Q. *Is there any limit to the number of low-calorie drinks I can have?*

A. I suggest you limit low-calorie drinks to three to four a day.

Q. *Why can't I cook with salt or add it to my food?*

A. Most people eat more than twice the salt or sodium they need. High sodium intake can cause fluid retention and has been implicated in high blood pressure. By reducing salt intake you'll experience fewer dieting plateaux (often due to temporary fluid retention) and perhaps prevent high blood pressure. Even without adding salt you'll be getting plenty of sodium in the foods you eat. Sodium is contained in many foods naturally and is frequently added to packaged foods by manufacturers for flavour and to retard spoilage. Even with my salt restriction, you'll still be getting 2000 to 2500 mg. of sodium per day. This amount is plenty; it also happens to be the level recommended by health and fitness experts.

Q. *Can't I use salt substitutes?*

A. Salt substitutes consist of either potassium or a combination of potassium and sodium. You don't need more potassium or sodium than you're getting from the diet. If you have a potassium deficiency, your doctor should supervise your diet. He may want to add potassium.

Q. *I miss the taste of salt. Isn't there some substitute I can use?*

A. Yes. Try out different herbs and spices. In any event, you'll soon get used to less salt. In fact, once you get used to less salt, salty foods will taste unpleasant and much too salty for you.

Q. *Can I drink herbal tea and spiced tea?*

A. Yes. These are fine and a great substitute for regular coffee and tea if you're trying to cut down on caffeine.

Q. *Can people with diabetes, high blood pressure, or heart trouble go on the Hilton Head Metabolism Diet?*

A. These people need to lose weight more than anyone else. However, they should definitely check with their doctor before going on this or any other diet, and he should supervise their programme. As diabetics lose weight, for example, they often need their insulin dosages modified.

Q. *What other benefits will I obtain from the Hilton Head Metabolism Diet besides losing weight?*

A. Well, you'll definitely be improving your metabolism and feeling more energetic. In addition, decreases in cholesterol, high blood pressure, and high blood sugar levels are typical.

Q. *Can I use steak sauce, tartare sauce, ketchup, and mustard?*

A. Definitely not. Avoid all of these unless specified in the menus. I have provided recipes for diet sauces for fish and prawns in Chapter 20.

Q. What if I don't like some of the foods in the Hilton Head Metabolism Diet?

A. *To be perfectly blunt, eat them anyway. I have provided substitution lists in Chapter 19, but the more you modify the diet, the less likely it is to work.*

Q. *Can I use honey as a substitute for sugar?*

A. No. Honey actually has more calories than sugar. It is definitely *not* a sugar substitute while dieting. Use dietetic sugar substitutes.

Q. *When you say I can eat mayonnaise in the Booster Phase, are you referring to diet mayonnaise?*

A. No. You can use regular mayonnaise. I'll specify dietetic when that's called for. I want you to be able to eat normal foods even while dieting.

Q. *Can I drink alcohol on the diet?*

A. No. Dieting and alcohol do not mix. Even an occasional glass of wine is out until you lose all your weight.

Q. *What can I substitute for alcohol at the cocktail hour or at a party?*

A. Soda water or Perrier on the rocks with a slice of lemon or lime makes a great 'Metabolism Cocktail'.

Q. *Some of the metabo-meals are more satisfying than others. Can't I switch them around or just eat the same one every night?*

A. Allow yourself a free choice for the metabo-meal once a week. Otherwise, stick strictly to my plan.

Q. *I really hate to eat breakfast. Can't I skip it and just have two metabo-meals, one in the afternoon and one in the morning?*

A. No. You must eat breakfast. The spacing of the meals is important for thermogenesis. If you're not used to breakfast, you'll soon become accustomed to it. I've had patients who absolutely hated to eat breakfast but now look forward to it.

Q. *I'm not losing weight on the Hilton Head Metabolism Diet as fast as my friend. What is wrong with me?*

A. Nothing is wrong with you other than metabolic suppression. Remember, people lose weight at different rates based on body size, how much weight they have to lose, gender, body fat, muscle, and past dieting history. Your metabolism won't change in a few days, especially if you scored very high on my Metabolism Suppression Test in Chapter 2. Have patience, and don't compare yourself with others. You are a unique individual and soon to become a *slim* unique individual.

Q. *I don't like bananas. Is this a problem on the diet?*

A. Yes, in a way it is. Bananas and tomatoes are excellent sources of potassium on any diet. Just make sure you eat the other potassium foods on the diet – potatoes, vegetables, and cantaloupe – without making further substitutions.

Q. *I don't ever eat meat. Can I still go on the Hilton Head Metabolism Diet?*

A. Certainly. You'll notice that since the diet is low in fat, beef is allowed only about two days a week. Simply substitute fish, chicken, or turkey on the beef days.

Q. *What if I get the flu? Should I stay on the diet?*

A. First of all, check with your doctor regarding the diet if you have a fever, flu, or serious illness. He may advise you to stick with the higher calorie Booster menus until you're feeling better. A simple cold should not interfere with the diet at all.

Q. *Is the Hilton Head Metabolism Diet okay for children and older people?*

A. The diet is fine for adolescents eighteen years of age and older. For younger children, check with your doctor. I usually don't advise young children to be put on the Low-cal menu plan. Rather, I put them on a two-week Booster, one-week Reentry programme until they lose their excess weight.

Older people should have no trouble with the diet.

Q. *What if I get up really late one day, say, 11:00 A.M.? Should I skip breakfast and make lunch the first meal of the day?*

A. No. Always eat breakfast, and always eat all the meals in order. If you get up at 11:00 A.M., eat breakfast, and then eat each of the rest of your meals a little bit later than usual.

Q. *What if I go off the diet one day? Should I skip a meal or eat less the next day?*

A. Definitely not. Never ever skip a meal. If you deviate from the diet, just go right back to it at the very next meal. If you feel the need to relieve some of your guilt through self-punishment, do it by exercising more the next day.

Q. *Have you personally ever had to diet?*

A. Yes. While I do not have a significant weight problem, I have gone on the Hilton Head Metabolism Diet to lose ten pounds. In fact, my wife and I went on the diet together. She lost thirty pounds and is now slim and trim. We both practise the rules of the Metabolism Plan – four balanced meals per day and exercise after two meals – to keep our metabolic furnaces burning brightly.

12

The Hilton Head Metabolism Exercise Plan

If you're like most people, you realize that exercise is good for you. You also realize that exercise helps burn extra calories. Unfortunately, knowing these facts and doing something about them are two different things.

Many people, especially overweight people, dislike physical activity. Mere mention of the word *exercise* sends them into a panic. You may even be trying to figure out how to go on the Hilton Head Metabolism Diet without exercising. Get those thoughts out of your head. I'm going to put you on the easiest exercise programme of your life. I'm also going to show you how to get the *most* benefit out of the *least* amount of exercise.

If you don't particularly care for exercise, don't feel bad about it. It's not easy when you're carrying around thirty or forty extra pounds. You just can't move your body as easily as someone who is at his ideal weight. However, if you start slowly and follow my plan, exercise will take on a new meaning.

One of my patients had never in her life been physically active before she came to me. She avoided walking, drove her car even to visit a friend only one block away, and wouldn't have been caught dead in an exercise class. After four weeks on my programme, she lost twenty pounds and was walking and biking every single day. Her husband and children couldn't believe it. She felt more energetic than she ever had and looked forward to her exercise. Now, two years later, she is keeping her weight off, walking every morning, and riding an exercise bicycle every evening. She recently told me, 'I can't believe the changes I've made. I can control my weight with just twenty minutes of exercise in the morning and twenty minutes in the evening. And the Metabolism Exercise Plan is easy. I don't have to strain. I go at my own pace and enjoy it. I actually look forward to my exercise. I feel like a new woman, inside and out.'

Maybe it's not that you dislike exercise, but you're just not disciplined enough to stick to it. How many times have you vowed, 'Today I'm going to start exercising. I'm fat, flabby, and out of shape. From now on I'm going to jog every day and work out at the health club three days a week'? So you start with an abundance of enthusiasm and the best of intentions. The first few days you push yourself to the limit. You forget that your muscles haven't been exercised in years. All of a sudden your body rebels. It's had it. You're sore all over. You can barely move. So you miss the next two days of exercise. And then it rains or the weather turns cold or you get too busy with the rest of your life. And that's the end of your exercise programme.

Forget about the past. You've been going about this the wrong way. You've been trying to do too much too soon, perhaps even doing the wrong kinds of exercise. You may have been told that it takes so much exercise to burn fat that it's just not worth it. Besides, you're not a world class marathoner and have no desire to become one.

Stop fretting and remember:

YOU DON'T HAVE TO SWEAT AND STRAIN TO BURN FAT.

That's right. You don't have to run to exhaustion or train for the Olympics to be slim and trim. Twenty minutes of moderate, 'fun' exercises twice a day is all that it takes.

Why Is Exercise Necessary?

'Why can't I diet without exercising?' patients ask me. 'I can lose weight without exercising. Besides I've heard that it takes hours to burn off just one pound.'

Well, if you want to increase your metabolism permanently, you must follow my exercise plan. You don't have to exercise for hours to get results. There are many misconceptions about physical activity and dieting. Forget everything you've ever heard and let me set you straight.

There are five reasons why exercise is *absolutely necessary* on the Hilton Head Metabolism Diet.

1. EXERCISE BURNS CALORIES

Whenever you are physically active, you burn additional calories. The best calorie-burning exercises are the simplest to do. Let's take walking as an example. Your jogging friends may tell you that walking is not strenuous enough to do you any good. That's nonsense! As far as calories are concerned, *walking is just as good as jogging*. In fact, walking burns as many calories as jogging. The number of calories your body burns during activity is related to the distance you travel, *not* how fast you go. This is so important for you to remember that I'm going to say it again. The number of calories your body burns is related to the distance you travel, *not* how fast you go.

This is great news for dieters. You burn about 100 calories a mile whether you walk or run. The only difference is that the runner is finished faster. It would take a walker about twenty minutes to complete his mile, while a runner could do it in less than half the time. So what? What's ten minutes? Why not relax and enjoy burning your 100 calories in twenty minutes?

Many people are astonished by these facts. It's difficult to believe that a runner is not burning a lot more calories than a walker per mile. Now, don't confuse cardiovascular fitness with burning calories. More strenuous exercise, aerobic exercise, does condition the heart and lungs better than less strenuous exercise. But let's take one thing at a time. Your goal is to burn fat and to burn as much of it as you can. We'll worry about your fitness level later, *after* you lose your weight.

Another important element involved in burning calories through physical activity is your body size. This is one instance in which being bigger is better. As a general rule, the bigger you are, the more calories you burn during exercise. Bigger refers to your height *and* weight. A 160-pound person burns 104 calories while walking one mile. A 240-pound person burns 154 calories in the same distance. The reason is simple. Try carrying an 80-pound weight for one mile, and you'll discover how much extra effort and energy it takes.

The best *Calorie Burners*, as I call them, are those exercises that require you to move your body from one point to another. These whole-body activities include walking, bicycling, swimming, rowing, and dancing. I'll have more to say about these later.

2. EXERCISE STIMULATES YOUR METABOLISM

As I said in Chapter 5, exercise stimulates your metabolism and keeps it stimulated even after the exercise is over. These metabolic after-effects can last several hours. So when you go for a mile walk, you're not just burning calories during that twenty-minute period. You're increasing the number of calories your body is burning for the next three or four hours. If you exercise twice daily, as

I advise, you'll be keeping your metabolic furnace burning strongly for most of the day.

3. EXERCISE AFTER MEALS DOUBLY STIMULATES YOUR METABOLISM

Now I'm going to let you in on an essential bit of information that most doctors don't even know. For years my patients would ask me, 'When is the best time of the day to exercise?' My answer was that as long as you exercised regularly, it really didn't matter when you did it. Well, now I know that it *does* matter, and it matters a lot.

There is an important link between dietary thermogenesis and exercise. You probably remember from Chapter 4 that thermogenesis, or the thermic effect, is the process by which your metabolism is stimulated after every meal you eat. Your metabolism burns calories at a faster rate for three to four hours after every meal. You should also be aware that *physical activity after meals doubles this thermic effect*. I can't stress to you enough how important this is.

By exercising *after* meals, you can increase the thermic stimulation of your metabolism from 25 per cent to as much as 50 per cent. Exercising after meals burns calories more efficiently than any other exercise schedule. You can't get as powerful an effect from your exercise or your meals in any other way. As you'll see, this mealtime-exercise connection is a basic underlying principle of my exercise plan.

4. EXERCISE DEVELOPS MUSCLE TISSUE

Certain exercises, which I refer to as *Muscle Firmers*, develop, tone, and firm muscle tissues. While they don't burn as much fat as the Calorie Burners, they are essential to metabolic efficiency. Your goal is to burn fat *and* develop muscle tissue.

Remember, the more muscle tissue, the higher your metabolism. You want to be as lean and as firm as you can get. If you just lose body fat without developing more muscle tissue, you won't be changing your metabolism nearly as much as you can. I want you to be burning every possible extra calorie. I want your body's furnace to be as finely tuned as possible.

I'm not saying you have to become a bodybuilder or that you have to be musclebound. You should be lean and firm. No more than 20 per cent of your body weight should be fat if you are a man, and no more than 25 per cent should be fat if you are a woman.

5. EXERCISE GIVES YOU ENERGY

In addition to the physiological effects of exercise on your metabolism, physical activity also gives you a terrific energy boost. Regular exercise makes you feel alive and in control of your life. It helps you keep the commitment and motivation to follow my dietary plan.

When you begin my exercise programme, you'll soon feel a strong sense of confidence in yourself. You'll be back in control of your body again. All of your bodily processes, not just your metabolism, will function better with regular, moderate exercise.

The Hilton Head Metabolism Exercise Plan

The Hilton Head Metabolism Exercise Plan is really quite simple and requires very little time. Before giving you your exercise prescription, let me describe the types of exercises that are required.

CALORIE BURNERS

The Calorie Burners, or whole-body exercises, are essential to your progress throughout the diet. These exercises burn the most calories and stimulate your metabolic rate on a day-to-day basis.

Calorie Burner exercises include the following:

1. WALKING. Walking at a moderate pace (one mile in about twenty minutes) is an excellent calorie burner. Walking outside in nice weather is pleasant, but remember you can also walk indoors. Whether you live in a small city apartment or a large country house, you can walk around your home and still get in a nice mile walk. Turn on the radio or play your favourite record or tape and walk along briskly with the music. Put on your headset, if you have one, and walk from room to room.

Walking around the house is also a great way to get household chores done. Empty wastepaper baskets as you go, or straighten the house by putting clothes, magazines, etc., in their proper places. Just keep moving!

What's great about walking as an exercise is that you don't need any special equipment. None, that is, except a good pair of walking shoes. The best shoes for walking, especially if you are overweight, are running shoes. I say they're the best, because they are both comfortable and, more importantly, they protect you from injury. Being overweight and under-exercised, you are a prime candidate for a foot, ankle, or knee injury. Because of the special arch and heel supports in running shoes, they are just what an overweight person needs for walking. There are many brands and styles to choose from. Go to a sporting goods store and explain that you want a good pair of running shoes for *walking*. If you have special arch or foot problems, consult your doctor. Take precautions *before* you begin my exercise plan, and you'll avoid injuries that may result in a frustrating setback.

If your doctor advises against walking because of foot, ankle, leg, knee, or back problems, don't worry about it. There are plenty of alternatives for you.

2. OUTDOOR BICYCLING. Bicycling at a moderate pace (two and a half to three miles in about twenty minutes) is also a great calorie burner. Many people enjoy cycling much more than walking. You don't need a fancy ten- or fifteen-speed machine. Most people who buy these end up using only one speed anyway. Any old bike that is in good working order will do.

Your cycling must be nonstop. If you live in a busy city and you must stop frequently for traffic, choose another Calorie Burner. If you have to contend with a lot of hills, you may also wish to choose another activity. If, on the other hand, the hills aren't too big, you might enjoy the challenge. Hills increase the effort required, and you end up burning more calories.

3. SWIMMING. If you have access to a pool, swimming is great exercise. Moderately paced swimming at a total rate of about 500 yards in twenty minutes is all that is necessary. It must be continuous swimming. A combination of floating, wading, and swimming doesn't count.

Many public facilities, health clubs, and local colleges have indoor pools that might be accessible to you. Swimming probably results in the fewest injuries of any exercise. It is perfect for anyone who cannot use walking as an exercise because of foot, knee, or back problems.

4. INDOOR EXERCYCLING. An indoor exercise bicycle is a good investment. Unfortunately, most people who own one have it stored in the basement, attic, or cupboard. It's not doing much good there.

I strongly recommend exercycling as a calorie-burning activity. It is convenient and can provide a method of exercise twelve months of the year regardless of where you live. It is especially useful if, because of climate or safety factors, your outside activities are limited. If a busy schedule is your problem, you can simply hop on the bike and be finished with your exercise in twenty minutes.

There are a great many varieties of these machines available, commonly costing between £85 and £350. I would suggest you look for one between £125 and £300 that has a speedometer, an odometer to measure how many miles you've travelled, and an adjustment to change the tension on the wheel (making it easier or more difficult to pedal). The fancy computerized versions are really not necessary.

Some exercycles have a flywheel rather than a regular bicycle wheel, making them quieter for home use. Shop around before making your decision which model to go for. Some types have a larger seat, which many people find more comfortable.

If exercycling seems boring to you, try watching television, listening to music, or reading while doing it.

5. REBOUNDING. You may not be familiar with this term, but rebounding is a new craze that's sweeping the United States. A rebounder (or bouncer) is a small (30 to 36 inches in diameter) round trampoline-like exerciser. You can jog in place on it, bounce on it, or dance on it. It's much better than walking or jogging in place, because you don't have the constant pounding of your body on the hard floor. And it's great fun besides. Just turn on the music and bounce away for twenty minutes. It's great for relieving tensions, and you'll feel like a kid again.

A rebounder can be purchased from your local sporting goods store for about £60.

6. ROWING (ROWING MACHINE). I must admit that I am partial to the rowing machine and use it for one of my exercise sessions each day. The beauty of the rowing machine is that it is both a Calorie Burner and a muscle-firming activity. Twenty minutes of rowing really gets your metabolism going. It also firms the muscles in your upper body, particularly in your arms and chest. It is really invigorating. You can close your eyes and imagine you're rowing along a sleepy lagoon with no cares in the world. Or, if you're feeling a bit competitive, you can imagine you're about to win an important race. Exercising should be fun and relaxing. Let yourself go. Use your imagination to take a twenty-minute 'vacation' from your daily routine. There's a bit of Walter Mitty in all of us.

You can purchase a good rowing machine for between £115 and £150. Make sure it's one that has a seat that moves forward and back as you row. This will help exercise your legs as well as your upper body.

7. SELF-CHOREOGRAPHED DANCING TO MUSIC. Actually, all that is required of a Calorie Burner exercise is for you to keep your body moving constantly for twenty minutes. If you're a little creative and enjoy dancing, just turn on your favourite music and let yourself go. Rock and roll, disco, classical, country and western, or even the fox trot will do. Make up your own steps as you go. Let your body move. Pretend you're choreographing a new Broadway musical, and try to come up with new routines.

If you enjoy dancing with a partner, grab your husband,

wife, friend, or just a broom, and let yourself go. Dancing every evening together can do wonders for your relationship.

YOUR DAILY ROUTINE

You must do the Calorie Burners twice each day. The timing of these exercises is *extremely* important. Because of the thermic effect, you must schedule these exercises *after* two of your four daily meals. Choose any two meals. Keep in mind, however, that you'll get maximum benefit if one of these meals is your dinner – the largest meal of the day. The larger the meal, the larger the metabolic boost you get from exercise.

Another important point is that you must wait twenty to thirty minutes after a meal before beginning your exercise. This allows the food enough time to stoke up your furnace. Then you'll really be supercharging your metabolism and burning the maximum number of calories.

Also remember that your exercise should last for twenty minutes each session. That's twenty minutes nonstop.

To summarize, here are your metabolic exercise guidelines:

DOs
1. *Do* wait twenty minutes after a meal to exercise.
2. *Do* keep your exercise going for at least twenty minutes.
3. *Do* plan to exercise after *two* of your four meals each day.

DON'Ts
1. *Don't* wait any longer than thirty minutes after a meal to begin exercising.

2. *Don't* strain; moderation is the key.
3. *Don't* miss a day.

PACING YOURSELF

To give you a better idea of how much exercise you should try to get into the twenty-minute exercise period, I'm providing you with an exercise chart. I've included walking, bicycling, swimming, exercycling, rebounding, rowing, and dancing to music. Moderation is the key. You're not trying to exhaust yourself, just to rev up your engine a bit. These are *not* aerobic exercises. You're not trying to increase your heart rate to a certain training level. All you're doing is increasing body movement for twenty minutes.

If you are way out of shape, you'll want to start slowly anyway. But, even as you lose weight and feel like you can push yourself, take it easy. I want you to establish a pattern of *regular, consistent, moderate* exercise that you will continue to enjoy for many years to come. Remember, faster is not better. The key is to aim for a regular, consistent distance and continue this pattern day after day after day.

The exercise chart on page 110 gives you specific guidelines to follow.

EXERCISE SCHEDULE

Plan to take your exercise after any two meals that seem convenient for your daily schedule. It's best to get into a solid routine so you're exercising after the same two meals every day. Some people prefer to exercise after breakfast and dinner. You may have to get up a little early, but it'll be worth it. If you're not a morning person, perhaps

Calorie Burners	Length of session	Approximate distance or rate
Walking	20 minutes	1 mile
Bicycling	20 minutes	2½–3 miles (8–9 miles per hour)
Swimming	20 minutes	500 yards (20 laps in 25-yard pool)
Exercycling	20 minutes	2½–3 miles (8–9 miles per hour)
Rebounding	20 minutes	A moderate, controlled pace (about 70–100 steps per minute)
Rowing (machine)	20 minutes	25–40 strokes per minute
Self-choreographed dancing	20 minutes	A moderate, controlled pace will do

exercising after a later meal might be better for you. Many of my patients who work take a brisk walk during their lunch break after eating. Others keep an exercycle at work for a twenty-minute ride after lunch. If you're a housewife, perhaps after breakfast and lunch might be the best time for you. Try to develop the habit of exercising after the same two meals; you're more likely to stick to a regular daily routine.

If you happen to miss one of your sessions, simply plan to do your exercise after one of the other meals that day. On a particularly hectic, busy day, you may end up exercising after dinner and after your metabo-meal. That's perfectly all right.

EXERCISE VARIATIONS

Should you do the same exercises every day or use some variety? The answer depends on whatever works best for you. Some people stick to exercise better if they do exactly the same routine day after day. Other people are easily bored with sameness and like a good variety.

All the Calorie Burners I've listed are equally good for you. I've equated all of the exercises in terms of calorie expenditure. If you stick to the twenty-minute distance or rates I've listed on the exercise chart, you can exchange one exercise for another and get exactly the same benefits.

Most of my patients choose two basic Calorie Burners for their daily exercise. These might be walking and exercycling, swimming and walking, or rebounding (bouncing) and dancing to music. Any two that you enjoy will do. You can use one of these for your first exercise period and the other for the second. Two or three times a week you may wish to throw in a different Calorie Burner for variety.

If you would prefer to use the same exercise twice a day, every day, that's perfectly okay. Several of my patients, especially those who live in the suburbs or out in the country, use walking as their daily after-meal activity. It is their exclusive exercise. They walk for two twenty-minute periods daily and enjoy it. My patients have come up with their own name for this activity – the *thermal walk*.

Your Personal Exercise Planner

Why not take this opportunity to plan your personal exercise routine? Take into consideration your family and work schedules and the times of day you're most likely to feel like exercising. Don't schedule exercise after a particular mealtime if there are likely to be a lot of interruptions.

Try to be realistic in your planning. What exercises do you enjoy? Which ones are you most likely to continue? Do you like a routine or variety?

Now fill in the following Personal Exercise Planner. Choose the two meals that would be best to follow up with exercise and the specific Calorie Burner exercises you'll be doing for the first week of the programme. Write in *walking, bicycling, swimming, exercycling, rebounding (bouncing), rowing,* or *self-choreographed dancing* under the appropriate two Meal columns for each day of the week.

Commitment and Time

I can hear you saying, 'All this talk about exercise is well and good, but I just don't have the time.' This is the most

Personal Exercise Planner

Day \ Meal	Breakfast	Lunch	Dinner	Metabo-Meal
Monday				
Tuesday				
Wednesday				
Thursday				
Friday				
Saturday				
Sunday				

frequent excuse I hear. Believe me, I realize you have to lead your normal life while dieting and exercising. And I realize that it's not always easy. But it's definitely not impossible.

First, look at your priorities. How important is it for you to lose weight and keep that weight off? If it *is* important, then you must take the time to do it right. *You* are the most important element of your life. That's right – you and your health and happiness. You must *make* the time. It might take some rearranging of your schedule, but you can do it. After all, I'm offering you a completely different way to lose weight permanently by burning more calories. This is not just another diet. This is the chance you've been waiting for. So don't hesitate. Make the time for yourself. Make the time to do this right, and you'll never have to worry about being overweight again.

Precautions – Exercise and Your Health

The exercise plan I've outlined is designed for use by people who are relatively healthy. If you have special health problems, such as heart trouble, high blood pressure, respiratory problems, or recurrent back pain, check with your doctor before going on my exercise programme. He may want to advise you and check your progress.

If you are over forty years of age, you should check with your doctor anyway, before going on an exercise programme. He may want to perform an EKG or a treadmill EKG (stress test) before you begin.

All Calorie Burners should be done at a moderate pace. If you are breathing so hard that you cannot carry on a normal conversation, you're overdoing it.

13
Muscle Firmers

When you get within ten pounds of your goal, it will be necessary to add the Muscle Firmer exercises. Before you get upset about adding more exercises, let me assure you that I'm not adding any extra exercise time. You'll still be exercising twice a day for twenty minutes each session. That's the total amount of time you'll ever need for exercise to keep you trim for ever.

Why Are Muscle Firmers Necessary?

Your goal at the beginning of your diet is to burn as many calories as possible. This is best accomplished by using the Calorie Burners as I have instructed. As a permanent way to raise metabolism, you must also develop as much muscle tissue as you can. While Calorie Burners develop some muscle tissue, their major function is to burn calories.

As you lose more weight, you must begin to add Muscle Firmers. These exercises don't burn as many calories, but they *do* firm, build, and tone muscle tissue. Remember, you want as much muscle tissue and as little body fat as possible. I'm not talking about being musclebound. I just want your body to be lean and hard rather than fat and flabby.

The basic idea behind the need for Muscle Firmers is

THE MORE MUSCLE,
THE HIGHER YOUR METABOLISM.

You should wait until you have lost all but ten pounds before beginning these exercises. Before then, concentrate on the Calorie Burner programme in Chapter 12, and forget about the Muscle Firmers. If you have only ten total pounds to lose, you can start the Muscle Firmers right away.

When Should You Do the Muscle Firmers?

The Muscle Firmers routine I am about to give you should be done three times a week during one of your regular after-meal, twenty-minute exercise periods. You'll simply be substituting a Muscle Firmer for one of your Calorie Burner exercises during one session on three days a week.

To give you a specific example, opposite is the exercise routine I set up for one of my patients when she was ten pounds from her ideal weight.

Remember, you're *not* adding exercise time, you are just exchanging a Calorie Burner for a Muscle Firmer during three exercise sessions a week.

It is extremely important for you to include these Muscle Firmers. In combination with the Calorie Burners, they constitute the best exercise for your metabolism.

What Are Muscle Firmers?

Muscle Firmers are a special set of muscle strengthening callisthenic exercises that I have put together for you. As you know, there are hundreds of different callisthenic exercises. Some are designed for flexibility, some for stretching muscles, and others for strengthening and developing muscle tissue.

Day	Breakfast	Lunch	Dinner	Metabo-Meal
Monday	Muscle Firmers		Exercycling	
Tuesday	Walking		Exercycling	
Wednesday	Muscle Firmers		Exercycling	
Thursday	Walking		Exercycling	
Friday	Muscle Firmers		Exercycling	
Saturday	Walking		Exercycling	
Sunday		Walking		Exercycling

If you've ever belonged to an exercise class or read books on body toning, you will realize that everyone seems to have his own system. Also, everyone claims that his system is better than anyone else's.

You must keep two things in mind about these different schools of thought. First, *you* need to exercise primarily to burn fat and speed up your metabolism. Most people who are regular attenders at exercise classes are not fat. In fact, most of them are slim and have been that way most of their lives. Oh, perhaps they put on four or five pounds occasionally, but they don't have the kind of weight problem you have. You need the special set of exercises that I'll give you. You need muscle development for your metabolism, not just flexibility and toning. People with weight problems need a very special exercise programme. Probably the best thing to do is forget everything you've ever been told about exercise. Let's clean the slate and start anew on your very *last* exercise plan.

A second important fact about callisthenics has to do with 'spot reducing'. Many exercise specialists will lead you to believe that certain callisthenics help reduce fat deposits in certain parts of your body. That is, special exercises will help you lose fat from your stomach, thighs or buttocks. I'm sorry to have to destroy another dieting/exercising myth, but this is simply not true. It's very misleading and can result in your doing the wrong kind of exercises.

When you do body toning exercises, you *can* tone, firm, and develop muscle, but you *cannot* get rid of fat in specific areas of your body. You burn fat by using the whole-body Calorie Burner exercises, and you firm up muscle with the Muscle Firmers. You burn more calories by walking than you do by going to an exercise class.

I'm not saying that toning exercises won't slim you in your arms, legs, stomach, or thighs. I'm just saying that the reason you're slimming is because muscles are firming, not because you're getting rid of fat. If you were to go to an exercise class for muscle toning without dieting, you would firm up a little, but you would still be overweight. The only exceptions to what I'm saying are the exercise classes that get your body moving, such as aerobic dancing or jazz exercises. These firm you *and* burn calories.

Just remember that my Muscle Firmers are the best for you. They develop muscle tissue, firm you up, and increase metabolism. For long-term success, however, you must also continue the Calorie Burners.

Muscle Firmers

The following are my twelve Muscle Firmers, which you should do three times a week. They should take no more than fifteen or twenty minutes to complete. Don't substitute any others. These, and only these, are designed for maximum metabolic increase. All of these exercises are for both men and women.

MUSCLE FIRMER No.1 – JUMPING JACK WARM-UPS

First of all, you need my jumping jack warm-up exercise to wake up all of your muscles. Stand straight up with your feet together and arms at your sides. Swing your arms upward until they're over your head. At the same time spread your feet apart sideways. Your arms should go up and your feet should spread apart in one continuous motion. Then return to the starting position by bringing your arms down and feet together in one smooth

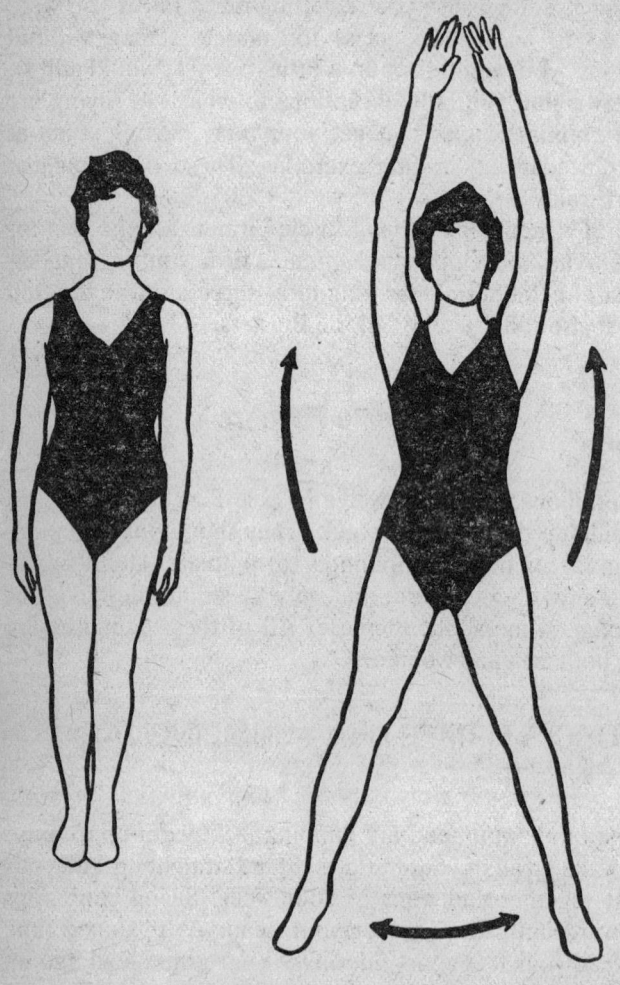

Muscle Firmer No. 1 – Jumping Jack Warm-ups

movement. Your pacing should be moderate. You're not in any big hurry.

REPETITIONS. Begin by doing ten and work up to twenty to twenty-five.

MUSCLE FIRMER No.2 – CURL-UPS

A curl-up is like a sit-up only it puts more stress on your stomach muscles and less on your back. Your stomach muscles must do all the work.

Lie flat on the floor with your legs bent at the knees and your feet flat on the floor. You must keep your legs bent at the knees. *Never do this exercise with your legs straight out.* Fold your hands across your chest. Sit up to a 30° angle and then lie down once again. You should curl your body up slowly, starting by moving your head forward and then bringing the rest of your body up. Come back down slowly. Avoid jerking your body up. Your rhythm should be smooth and slow. Unlike a sit-up, you do not want to bring your body up all the way to a sitting position. Sit up about halfway (30°), and then go back down again.

REPETITIONS. Try to do anything from one to six at first, and over a series of weeks try to increase gradually to thirty. If you can only do one or two at first, don't worry about it. Do what you can and increase gradually.

MUSCLE FIRMER No.3 – PUSH-UPS

Push-ups are great for strengthening your forearms, the backs of your upper arms, your chest, and stomach. Two types of push-ups are available – the beginner's and the advanced.

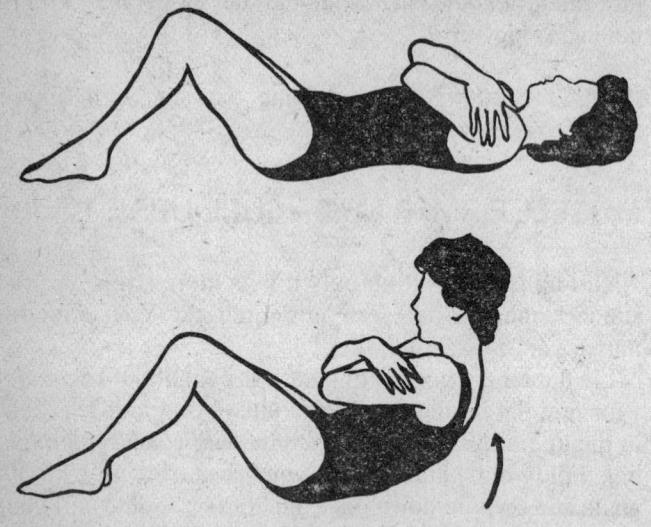

Muscle Firmer No. 2 – Curl-ups

The *beginner's push-up* is designed for people who have not exercised in a long time. Many women prefer this type of push-up. If these are easier for you than the advanced ones, you can use these exclusively even after you get in shape. Lie facedown on the floor with your legs together. Place your hands, palms down, on the floor at about shoulder width. Keeping your knees and toes in contact with the floor, push your upper body off the floor, straightening your arms. Make sure you keep your back straight. The important part of the beginner's push-up is to keep your knees on the floor the whole time.

REPETITIONS. Begin your first few sessions by doing between one and six. Your eventual goal should be to do between twenty and thirty at a time. Proceed slowly.

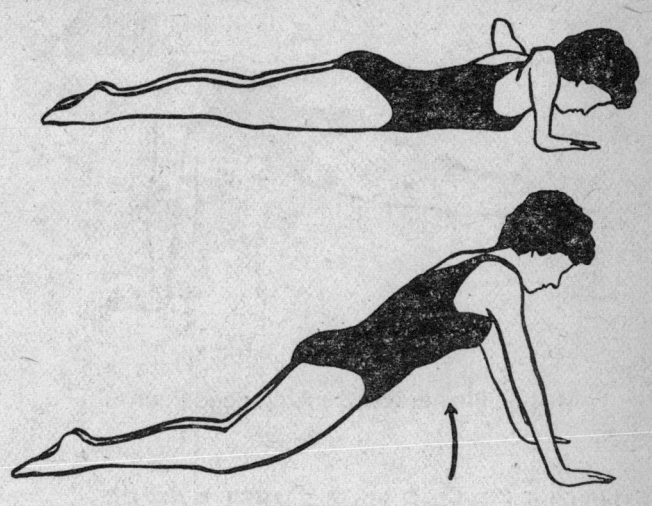

Muscle Firmer No. 3 – Beginner's Push-ups

The *advanced push-up* is similar, but much more difficult to do. Lie on the floor facedown, with your legs together. Place your hands, palms down, on the floor at about shoulder width. Keeping your toes and hands in contact with the floor, push your body up off the floor, straightening your arms. Lower your body by bending your arms until your chest is about one inch from the floor. Then push yourself up again.

REPETITIONS. Begin the first few sessions by doing between one and six. Your goal should be twenty-five to thirty. Proceed slowly. If you can only do one or two of these, start out the first few sessions with the beginner's push-up.

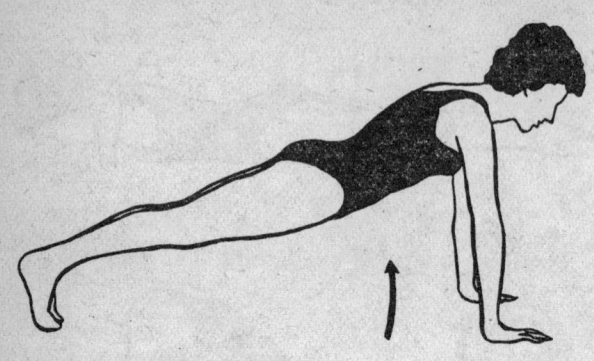

Muscle Firmer No. 3 – Advanced Push-ups

MUSCLE FIRMER No.4 – HEEL RAISES

This exercise will strengthen your leg muscles. Stand up straight with your feet about six inches apart. Keep your arms by your sides. Raise up on your toes, bringing your heels off the floor. Then lower your heels back again.

REPETITIONS. Start by doing ten and work up to twenty to thirty.

MUSCLE FIRMER No.5 – SIDE LEG LIFTS

These side leg lifts are great for the upper part of your legs. Lie on your right side with your right arm extended in line with your body and your left palm on the floor in front of your chest. Lift your left leg about two feet in the air. Then lower it. After twenty repetitions, turn over and repeat the exercise with your right leg.

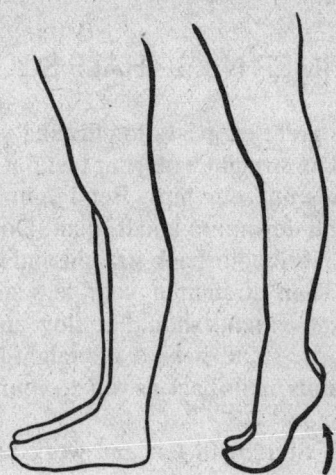

Muscle Firmer No. 4 – Heel Raises

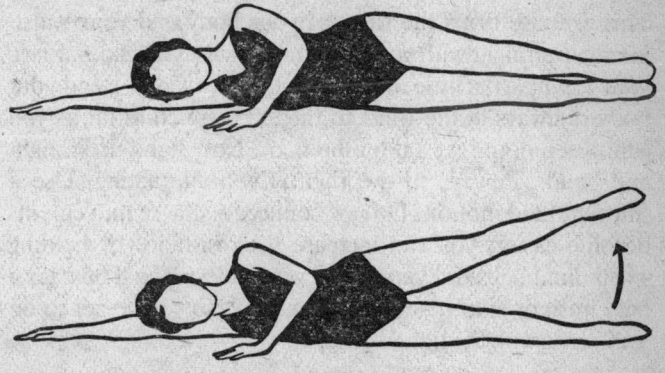

Muscle Firmer No. 5 – Side Leg Lifts

REPETITIONS. Start with ten for each leg and work up to twenty to twenty-five.

MUSCLE FIRMER No.6 – HALF SQUATS

Half squats are great exercises for firming your legs and buttocks. Stand up straight with your feet flat on the floor. Place your hands on your hips. Bend your knees about halfway, and sink down into a half squat. Do not bend all the way down. Keep your back straight and your feet flat on the floor. Then straighten your legs and stand up straight. Your movements should be slow and smooth. If you feel unsteady, stand behind a straight-backed chair and rest your hands on its back as you do your half squat.

REPETITIONS. Start with ten and work up to twenty-five.

MUSCLE FIRMER No.7 – SIDE BENDS

This exercise firms the sides of your body and your waist. Stand up straight with your arms hanging by your sides. Place your feet apart, a little more than shoulder width. Bend your body sideways at the waist to the left. Stretch as far as you can. Keep both feet flat on the floor. Now stand up straight and bend sideways to the right. Keep alternating. Use a smooth, fluid motion. Do not bounce. As these movements become easier, you can increase the resistance by holding small dumbbells or even tins of vegetables. You'll be eating only fresh or frozen vegetables anyway, so you've got to do something with the tinned ones.

REPETITIONS. Start with ten on each side and work up to twenty.

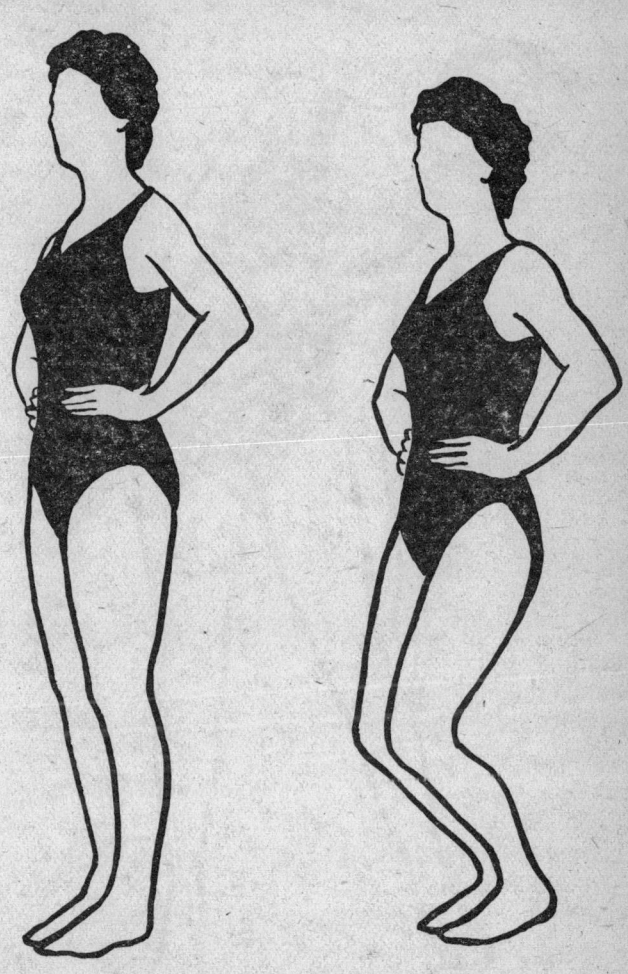

Muscle Firmer No. 6 – Half Squats

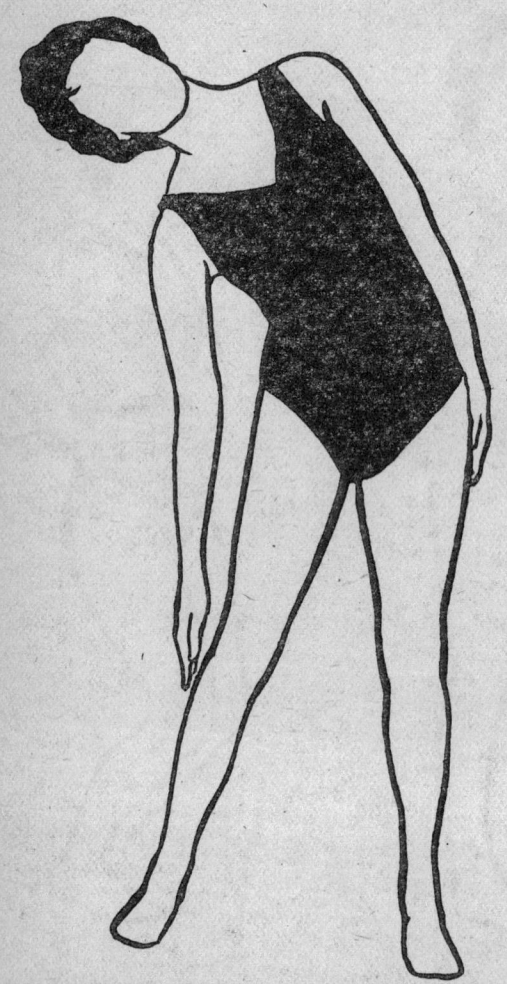

Muscle Firmer No. 7 – Side Bends

MUSCLE FIRMER No.8 – ARM CIRCLES

If you have flabby arms, these exercises will firm your arm muscles. Stand up straight, with your arms extended straight out to both sides of your body. Keeping your arms straight, rotate both arms in small clockwise circles. After twenty repetitions, repeat in a counterclockwise motion.

REPETITIONS. Start with ten in each direction and work up to twenty-five.

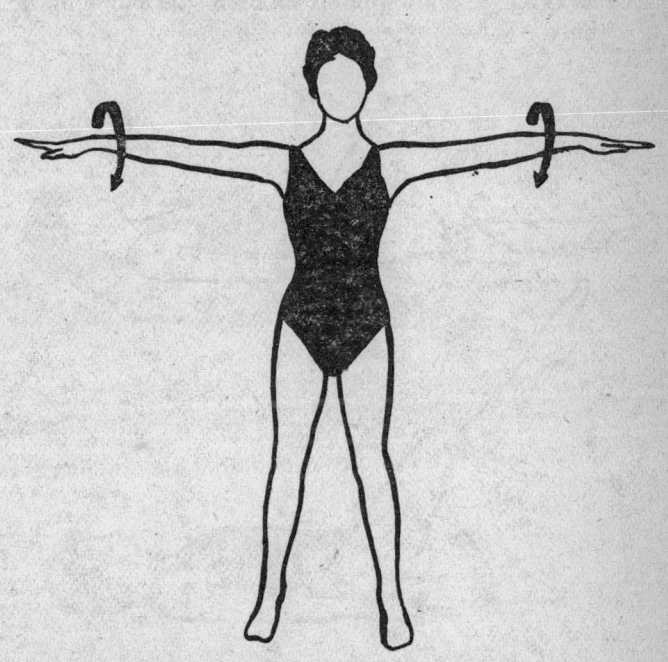

Muscle Firmer No. 8 – Arm Circles

MUSCLE FIRMER No.9 – LEG RAISES

This exercise is especially good for firming the thighs and upper legs. Lie flat on your back, with your body fully extended. Place your hands straight along your sides. Bend one leg at the knee, keeping your foot flat on the floor. Raise the extended leg in the air until it is at a 45° angle. Bring it back down and repeat ten to fifteen times. Then repeat, using the other leg. It is essential that you bend one leg during this exercise to take the strain off your lower back.

REPETITIONS. Start with six on each side and work up to twenty.

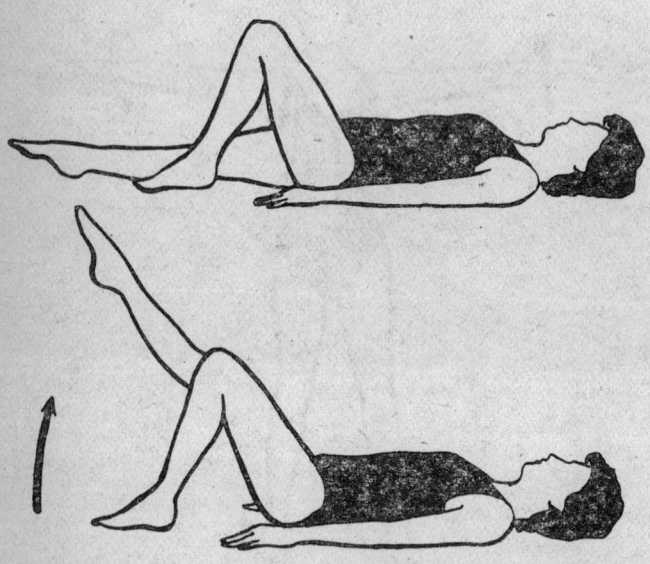

Muscle Firmer No. 9 – Leg Raises

MUSCLE FIRMER No.10 – READY, STEADY, GO

The ready, steady, go exercise strengthens your upper arms, buttocks, chest, and hips. Get down on the floor as if you're a runner squatting down to start a race. Both arms should be extended, supporting the upper part of your body. Your palms should be flat on the floor. One leg should be extended behind you, and the other leg should be bent slightly at the knee and drawn up under your chest. Don't bend your knee totally. Keep your arms straight and alternate the position of your legs. Bring one leg up and push the other back. Keep alternating in a smooth motion.

REPETITIONS. Start with ten and work up to twenty-five.

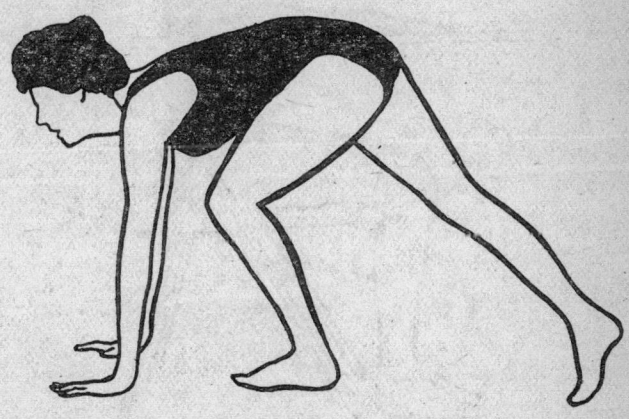

Muscle Firmer No. 10 – Ready, Steady, Go

MUSCLE FIRMER No.11 – ARM STRENGTHENERS

To firm and develop your arm muscles, you'll need a little help from a table or desk. Sit in a chair in front of a heavy desk or table. Place both hands, palms down, on top of the table. Press down with about 60 to 70 per cent of your strength. Hold this tension for six seconds. Then put your palms under the table as if you were going to pick it up.

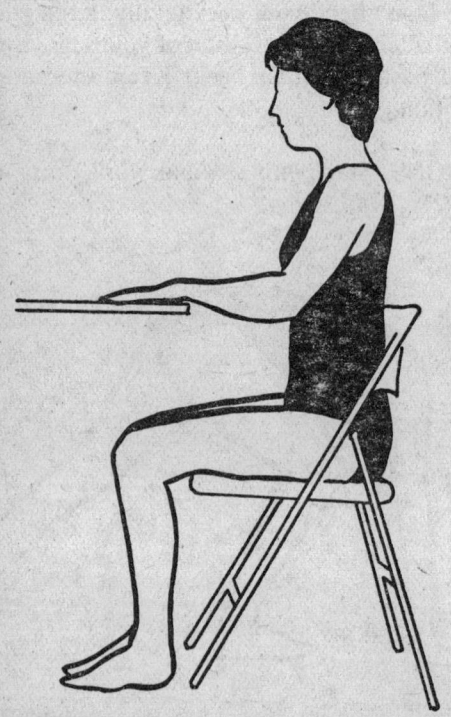

Muscle Firmer No. 11 – Arm Strengtheners

Press your hands upwards, using about 60 to 70 per cent of your strength. Hold the tension for six seconds and then release. Make sure you are breathing comfortably. Do not hold your breath during this exercise.

REPETITIONS. This isometric exercise requires only one repetition for maximum benefit.

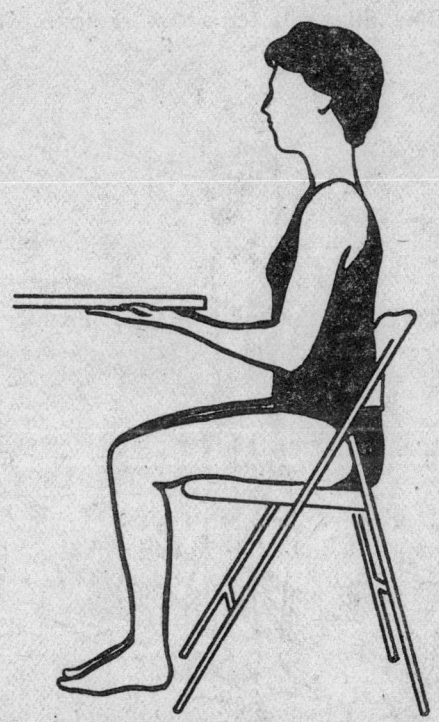

MUSCLE FIRMER No.12 – SHUFFLE

The shuffle is great for your buttocks and legs. Stand up straight, but bend your knees slightly. Put one foot slightly in front of the other so the toe of one foot is near the heel of the other. Shuffle your feet back and forth in a rapid motion. Make sure you keep your feet flat on the floor and your knees slightly bent. Make sure you shuffle. Don't bounce.

REPETITIONS. Start with ten and work up to twenty or twenty-five.

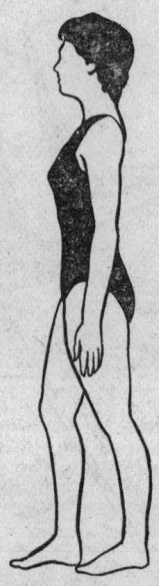

Muscle Firmer No. 12 – Shuffle

As an easy reference, I'm providing you with the chart on page 136 to use as your Muscle Firmer guide. You can refer to it quickly for the sequence of exercises.

Increasing Resistance

As you get used to these exercises, you'll find that they will become easier and easier. You'll be able to do more repetitions of each one. However, repetitions alone will not build muscle tissue. You must try to increase the resistance. That is, you must try to make the exercises more difficult.

There is usually enough resistance while doing curl-ups and push-ups. You can add resistance to the side leg lifts and the leg raises by wearing heavy shoes during the exercises. After many weeks of repetition, you could also add ankle weights to make these exercises harder. (You can buy ankle weights in most sporting goods stores.) When doing the arm circles and side bends, you can hold small dumbbells, books, or tins of food.

Just remember to start slowly. At first, do only as many repetitions as you can without straining. Go very, very slowly. Increase the repetitions by only two or three each week. Go even slower if you have to. These exercises are important, but not important enough for you to hurt yourself.

Muscle Firmers

Exercise	Repetitions for beginners	Repetitions after several weeks
1. Jumping jacks	10	20–25
2. Curl-ups	1–6	30
3. Push-ups	1–6	20–30
4. Heel raises	10	20–30
5. Side leg lifts	10 (each leg)	20–25 (each leg)
6. Half squats	10	25
7. Side bends	10 (each side)	20 (each side)
8. Arm circles	10	25
9. Leg raises	6	20
10. Ready, steady, go	1	1
11. Arm strengtheners	10	25
12. Shuffle	10	20–25

Hints to Remember

- Start with the Calorie Burners – twice a day after meals.
- Add Muscle Firmers three days a week when you get to within ten pounds of your goal.
- Each exercise session should last twenty minutes.
- Progress slowly.
- Enjoy yourself as you exercise.

14

Questions and Answers about the Hilton Head Metabolism Exercise Plan

These are the most commonly asked questions about my exercise plan:

Q. *I live in a very cold climate. How can I walk when it's so cold and snowy?*

A. Walking in very cold weather actually speeds up your metabolism and burns more calories. If it's simply too cold, snowy, or rainy to walk outside, I have provided several indoor alternatives. These include walking around the house, dancing to music, exercycling, indoor rowing, or rebounding (bouncing).

Q. *Why haven't you mentioned skipping or jogging in place?*

A. While these exercises are good for developing cardiovascular fitness, they are potentially harmful to anyone who is overweight. The repeated jolting of your body against the floor puts undue strain on your legs, knees, ankles, and feet. If you have any kind of back trouble, you should be particularly careful of these exercises.

Q. *I am fifty-five years old, forty pounds overweight, and haven't exercised in years. Are there any precautions I should take before going on your exercise plan?*

A. Yes. You definitely should consult your doctor before starting any exercise programme, especially at your age and weight. He may want you to take a treadmill electrocardiogram test (often called a stress test) to check your heart. He also may want you to start very slowly, perhaps walking only a quarter or half mile at a time at first until you become more accustomed to exercise.

Q. *I belong to an aerobic dancing class and attend on three days a week. Could I eat my lunch thirty minutes before class on these days and count this as one of my metabolism exercise sessions?*

A. Definitely, yes. This would be a fine idea. The more you can incorporate my plan into your regular routine, the better.

Q. *Is it all right to do the same type of exercise twice a day? I find it easier to hop on my indoor exercise bike after meals every day.*

A. It's perfectly okay to use the same exercise each day. Some people are more consistent if they keep up exactly the same exercise routine. Other people need more variety in their lives and like to vary the exercises. Either way will do.

Q. *Would you suggest that I do your exercises alone or together with someone else?*

A. Again, it depends on your personality. If you are a 'people' person, then by all means find an exercise partner. Couples who are dieting together often enjoy exercising together. They enjoy having someone to talk to. On the other hand, some people use their exercise times to relax and 'get away from it all'. They prefer to be alone during exercise, so they can unwind, meditate, or let their minds wander.

Q. *I lead a very active life. I'm on the go all the time, with ferrying the children, shopping, and running errands. Why do I need to exercise after all this activity?*

A. I'm sorry to say that your 'running around' all day counts very little as a calorie-burning activity. For physical activity to burn fat, it must be continuous and timed right (e.g. *after* meals). Your stop-and-go activities are not enough.

Q. *I'm so worn out at the end of my working day that I don't have enough energy for your exercise plan. How can I exercise when I'm exhausted?*

A. Probably the most frequent complaint I hear from my patients, in addition to being overweight, is a lack of energy. My diet and exercise programme will give you more energy than you've had in years. After a busy day, exercise will give you *more* energy even though you may feel exhausted. If you exercise for twenty minutes after dinner, I promise that you won't fall asleep on the couch watching television as you usually do. You'll feel rejuvenated. Remember that most of the fatigue you feel after work may be mental rather than physical.

Q. *Although I am about twenty pounds overweight, I jog three miles every day at an eight-minute-per-mile pace. Do I have to schedule my run after a meal?*

A. I do not recommend strenuous exercises after meals unless they occur thirty minutes after a very light meal such as the metabo-meal. Schedule your jogging for any time you like. However, I would still suggest my thermic exercises after two of your four meals. These should be moderately paced and not strenuous.

Q. *When you say I should exercise twenty to thirty minutes after a meal, is that the length of time after the beginning or end of my meal?*

A. You should estimate the time from the end of your meal.

Q. *What if I feel like exercising more than twenty minutes after a meal?*

A. If you have the time and the inclination, by all means, walk or cycle a little further. Just don't overdo it.

Q. *What if I'm eating dinner out and can't start my exercise until one or two hours after a meal?*

A. The optimum time for exercise is twenty minutes after a meal, but you can wait as long as one hour. If two hours have elapsed, I would suggest that you exercise after your next meal. However, if it's your last meal of the day and you've only had one other exercise time, then you should exercise, regardless of the time.

Q. *Will your exercises get rid of cellulite in my thighs and hips?*

A. Probably the biggest hoax perpetrated on the American public is the concept of cellulite. Cellulite is supposed to be a special, dimply kind of fat that women get on their hips and thighs. The truth of the matter is that cellulite is simple normal, everyday fat. It's the same kind of fat that you have in the rest of your body. Some people inherit a tendency to have more fat in the lower portion of their bodies. The lumpy, dimpling effect is simply caused by the size and spacing of fat cells. Such fat can only be removed by dieting. Exercise will firm muscles in the thighs and hips, but dieting will burn the fat.

15

Maintaining Your Weight Loss

Once you've lost all your excess weight, you'll not only have got rid of body fat, but also reprogrammed your metabolism. It's been reprogrammed in two ways. First, your basal metabolic rate will be higher. That means that you'll be burning calories at a higher rate even when you're resting. Second, and what I consider even more important, your metabolism has become more efficient. It is more responsive during the day, increasing much more than it ever did in response to such factors as meals, exercise, and climate variation. Your thermostat has been repaired and is functioning at full throttle.

This increased efficiency is well illustrated by changes in your metabolic reactions to meals. The thermic effect you get from meals definitely will be increased. A major reason is that you're eating four meals instead of three, adding an extra metabolic boost you weren't getting before. If you had been skipping some meals (breakfast, for example), the change would be even more pronounced. Also, you've lost fat and gained muscle. If you remember what I said earlier, fat people experience a thermic increase after meals of only 3 to 9 per cent. Fit and trim people can have a thermic effect that raises their metabolism by as much as 25 per cent. And that's a 25 per cent increase *four* times a day, now that you're eating a metabo-meal.

Let me give you an actual case example. A thirty-nine-year-old male patient of mine who is five feet eleven inches tall lost twenty-five pounds on the Hilton

Head Metabolism Diet. He followed my programme to the letter. A few weeks after his weight loss, he asked me to calculate exactly how many extra calories he was burning just from his body's increased responsiveness to the thermic effect. Before his weight loss, he typically ate no more than two or three large meals a day and rarely exercised. During the time he was on the Hilton Head Metabolism Diet, he ate four meals every day and exercised twice daily as prescribed. He lost his twenty-five pounds of fat and became lean and trim. Based on his metabolic suppression before the diet, he was getting about 25 calories per day extra benefit from the thermic effect. Because he is thinner and more solid and is eating four meals each day, he now receives a 100-calorie benefit from the thermic effect. That's almost 700 calories per week more than he was burning before the Hilton Head Metabolism Diet. And those calories are being burned without his even trying to burn them. All he has to do to get these free calories is make sure he eats four meals a day! That's not even counting the extra calories he is burning because of exercise after meals, the after-effects of exercise on metabolism, the nutritional composition of his meals, and the increase in his lean body mass.

All of these factors taken together account for 500 calories more per day now being burned. Five hundred calories a day more without much extra effort. That adds up quickly – 3500 calories a week, 15,000 calories a month.

How to Maintain Your 'Gains'

After you've lost your weight, you must make sure you keep up the gains you've made in improving your metabolism. Such gains don't occur overnight, so even after you've lost weight, you'll still be making metabolic improvements. Your metabolism will need more time to be reprogrammed, especially if you only had ten or fifteen pounds to lose. It may take several weeks to completely recondition your body's furnace. In fact, through my exercise plan you'll continue to develop muscle tissue even after you've lost your fat. So, month after month, as you're developing more muscle, your metabolism will be increasing even more.

When you finish the Reentry Phase of the diet, the only part of my plan you'll be changing is the number of calories you'll be eating. To maintain your ideal weight after the diet, you should simply eat normally. You don't have to diet, and you don't have to be overly strict with your calories. Generally speaking, women should be able to eat between 2000 and 2500 calories per day and maintain their weight. That's if you've done what I've told you and *if* you continue to do so. Men should be able to eat between 2500 and 3000 calories after the diet. It is very likely that before the diet you would have gained a considerable amount of weight on this number of calories. Now things are different. You should be able to maintain a perfect weight eating this amount of food.

I'm not saying that you have to count calories. An intake of 2000 to 2500 calories a day is plenty of food to eat, and you shouldn't have trouble sticking to this level. Besides, your appetite will be under better control after the diet. The bodily mechanisms that control hunger function best when you are at your ideal weight. Regular exercise also keeps you feeling less hungry.

Even though you've lost weight and are eating a normal amount of food again, you must protect yourself from slipping back into metabolic suppression. I never want you to be fat again. Never! Say that out loud as enthusiastically as you can:

'I WILL NEVER BE FAT AGAIN!'

Doesn't that sound great? It's not just an empty promise either. You can do it. You *can* keep that metabolism burning strongly.

To keep your metabolism at its maximum efficiency, follow these guidelines *for the rest of your life:*

MUSTS

1. *You must* eat four meals every day.
2. *You must* never eat between meals.
3. *You must* exercise after two meals a day.
4. *You must* perform my Muscle Firmers three times per week.
5. *You must* eat nutritionally well-balanced meals.

All of these principles must be incorporated into your lifestyle. They must become a permanent part of your day-to-day routine. After a while, you'll do them naturally, without thinking. It's like brushing your teeth. You don't really have to make a decision each morning about brushing your teeth. You've been so well conditioned, you just do it. It should be the same with your eating and exercise schedule.

NUTRITIONAL GUIDELINES

If you keep up doing the Calorie Burners and Muscle Firmers and eat four meals every day, you can eat just about anything you want. Remember, four meals a day *for sure*, but four meals a day *only*.

When I say you can eat just about anything, I mean it. You don't have to give up anything. Now, I'm not saying you can eat two gallons of ice cream a day, but you can eat ice cream and sweets occasionally. By 'occasionally', I'm talking about having a medium bowl or cone of ice cream or a couple of doughnuts or biscuits three to four times a week. Moderation is the key with sweets, primarily because they are not healthy for you.

Just keep in mind the optimum nutritional balance that I mentioned earlier.

15%-20%	Protein (chicken, fish, cheese, nuts, lean beef, milk)
55%	Carbohydrates (fruits, vegetables, potatoes, cereal, bread)
25%-30%	Fat (margarine, salad oil, beef, chicken, cheese, nuts, peanut butter)

If you are maintaining your weight on 2500 calories, this means that about 500 of these calories should be protein, 1400 carbohydrate, and 600 fat. That's the proportion that will keep your metabolism well tuned.

You can spread these calories out in your four meals any way you wish. One possibility that I often suggest is as follows:

Breakfast	400 calories
Lunch	800 calories
Dinner	900 calories
Metabo-meal	400 calories

This provides a good balance and gives you an adequate thermic effect after each meal.

You may wonder how you're going to eat so much after dieting. Don't worry. Remember, I told you your system is now ready for it.

To give you a little more direction, I suggest you follow my nutritional guidelines below:

1. Limit your intake of beef to no more than two to three times per week.

2. Watch your sodium intake.

3. Limit your intake of sugar, colas, and sweets.

4. Limit your intake of animal fat. Switch permanently to low-fat milk and vegetable oil margarine.

5. Add high fibre and bran foods to your diet.

6. Continue to eat *fresh* fruits and vegetables. Frozen ones will do as a substitute. Avoid tinned vegetables.

7. Trim excess fat off meats.

8. Grill, bake, and boil rather than fry.

9. Use less white sugar, brown sugar, honey, and syrups.

10. Eat fewer sweets, soft drinks, ice cream, biscuits and cakes.

11. Limit your intake of salty foods such as potato chips, pretzels, salted nuts, and pickled foods.

How You Can Monitor Your Progress

You should constantly monitor yourself to make sure you are keeping your metabolism high. Although there is no simple way for you to measure your metabolism without special equipment, you can get a fairly good estimate of your progress by evaluating your *weight*, *body measurements*, and *habits*.

WEIGHT

You must keep track of your body weight to make sure it stays within an ideal range. Once you've lost your excess weight, you should weigh *twice* each week. Weigh in the morning before breakfast every Monday and Friday.

You should expect normal fluctuations in your weight from day to day. Variations of one to three pounds are perfectly natural and should not bother you. These slight variations are the reason I recommend against your weighing every day. Twice a week is plenty after you've lost your weight. It's too easy to become obsessed with your weight if you hop on the scales every day.

BODY MEASUREMENTS

You should take your body measurements once every other week. Every other Monday morning you should measure in addition to weighing yourself.

If you are a woman, you should measure your *abdomen* and *thigh* as follows:

Abdomen	– Measure your abdomen at the level of the navel, keeping the tape measure as straight as you can.
Thigh	– Measure your right thigh one inch below where your leg meets your buttocks.

If you are a man, you only have to take the abdomen measurement.

These body measurements can give you a good idea of your lean body mass and body fat content. I have calculated the upper limits of these abdomen and thigh measurements for you. For women to maintain an ideal body fat content of 25 per cent or less, they must not exceed the abdomen and thigh measurements I have listed below.

Women
Maximum abdomen and thigh measures for ideal body composition

Height/Weight Category	Abdomen	Thigh
4'6"–4'11" (90–120 lb)	28"	20"
5'0"–5'5" (95–130 lb)	29"	21"
5'6"–5'9" (114–145 lb)	30"	22"
5'10"–6'1" (130–165 lb)	31"	23"

First, find your height and weight category. Next, look to the right of this category for your maximum abdomen and thigh measurements. For example, if you are five feet five inches tall and weigh 120 pounds, your abdomen should be twenty-nine inches or less, and your thigh should be twenty-one inches or less. If they are, it is likely that you are keeping your muscles firm and your body fat low. If you start to exceed these limits, you'd better watch it.

You're letting your metabolism slip back to its old sluggish pattern again.

Men only need to keep track of the abdomen measurement. The chart below lists the maximum abdominal measurements for men of different weights.

Men
Maximum abdomen measure for ideal body composition

Height/Weight Category	Abdomen
5'2"–5'4" (120–140 lb)	30"
5'5"–5'10" (141–160 lb)	32"
5'11"–6'2" (161–190 lb)	34"
6'3"–6'6" (191–225 lb)	36"

Find your weight category and check the abdomen measurement associated with it. Your abdomen must measure this number of inches or less for you to keep your body fat at 15 per cent or less – the ideal for men.

HABITS

Once every week, preferably on Sunday evening or Monday morning, you should schedule a time when you can sit quietly and review your habits. Think back over the past week and ask yourself these questions:

1. Did I eat four meals every day? If not, why not?

2. Did I do my Calorie Burner exercises after two meals every day? If not, why not?

3. Did I do my Muscle Firmer exercises three times this week? If not, why not?

4. Were my meals nutritionally well balanced? If not, why not?

Do a little self-confrontation. Be honest. If you didn't stick to the programme, try to find out why. Were you on holiday? Did you have guests? Were you upset? Try to figure out a way to keep on my plan regardless of these factors. Learn from your mistakes. Don't let them discourage you. Ask yourself, 'If that happens again, how can I deal with it better? How can I make sure I stick to the programme in spite of stress, other people, travel, or special occasions?'

Then think about the week to come. Do you see any obstacles to your meals or exercises? Do a little constructive planning. If Thursday is going to be a busy day, make sure you get your exercise in early, after breakfast. And make sure you plan to take the time for your four meals. Remember your priorities. *You and your new trim body are important, very important.*

Remember:

- Weigh twice a week.
- Measure twice a month.
- Review habits once a week.

The Metabolism Checklist

Based on your regular self-evaluations, keep a record of your success by using the Metabolism Checklist on page

153. It allows you to summarize quickly weight, measurements, and habit information for continued reference. Write in your weight and measurements as you take them. Look up the weight charts in Chapter 7 if you need to check your ideal weight. Check your body measurements against my charts in this chapter. Don't allow yourself to go over my maximum measurements for your weight. Give yourself a + or a − for the habit categories of Meals, Calorie Burners, and Muscle Firmers. You've either been doing them or you haven't. If not, get busy.

Maintain these records continuously to make sure you keep your metabolism fired up.

What to Do If You Put on a Few Pounds

If you get on the scales and are more than three pounds overweight, don't panic. The first thing to do is ask yourself if you've been keeping on my programme. If not, where have you gone wrong?

Next, switch immediately to my Reentry meal plan until you've lost the excess weight. If you have put on more than five pounds, go to the Booster menus, and then switch to the Reentry meals when you are one or two pounds from your goal. Usually the Reentry menu plan for a week or two is sufficient to get your desired weight back. *Never allow your weight to get more than five pounds above your ideal weight.*

With your new metabolism, your weight won't be increasing as quickly or easily as before. Any increases that do occur will be gradual and controllable. Your days of gaining five to ten pounds over a weekend are over.

The Metabolism Checklist

Category	Goal	Weeks					
		1	2	3	4	5	6
Weight	Ideal for height (see Chapter 7)						
Abdomen	Ideal for weight (see chart in this chapter)						
Thigh	Ideal for weight (see chart in this chapter)						
Meals	4 each day						
Calorie Burners	Twice daily after meals						
Muscle Firmers	3 times per week						

16

Keeping Your Motivation High

Keeping yourself motivated is an important key when you are trying to lose weight. Since the Hilton Head Metabolism Diet is based on such a revolutionary new concept, motivation is usually not a problem. Once you understand my approach and get started on the diet, you will feel a sense of enthusiasm and motivation that will carry you through to your goal. And remember, your goal is not simply to lose weight. Your goal is to change your metabolism permanently so you will be able to eat normally, maybe for the first time in your life. This notion of really being able to change your body chemistry for ever will keep you on the programme day after day.

Being human, you may experience brief lapses in motivation from time to time. This is especially true if you have a lot of weight to lose. Here are some hints on how to keep your motivation high.

Keeping Your Goals in Mind

The number one thing you must guard against is *impatience*. You will want your excess weight to disappear in a few days. Just like many of life's challenges, dieting requires time and patience. You must give it a chance to work.

By keeping your eventual weight goal in mind, you can ward off these feelings. Start by figuring out the specific reasons why you are trying to lose weight and to lose it for ever. Consider both the short-term and long-term future. What are the advantages to *you*, personally, to lose weight?

To help you answer this question, let's imagine you have already lost your excess weight. You are slim and trim and have been that way for one full year. You feel totally in control of your weight. You are able to eat normally without gaining weight. As you think this pleasant thought, make a list of as many advantages of being slim and trim as you can think of. Try to make them personally relevant.

Write your list on an index card, so you can keep it handy. One of my patients came up with the following list of pluses:

- I would feel more attractive.
- I would feel proud of myself and have more self-confidence.
- I would be less moody and not as likely to feel resentful, sensitive, angry, and depressed.
- I would be able to wear smaller sized and more stylish clothes.
- I would feel more outgoing and be more socially active.
- I would have a more enjoyable sex life and not be ashamed of my body.
- I would be more physically active and more involved in recreational activities.
- I would live longer and lessen the likelihood of being disabled by a stroke or heart attack.
- I would serve as a good example to others, particularly my children.

Keep this list in a prominent place at home. Put it where you will see it every day. Every few days during the diet, and especially when your motivation is low, read the list over very carefully. Read each item and think about it. Then pick one or two for more intense consideration.

Let's suppose you pick the one about your clothes fitting better. Now close your eyes and imagine that you have already lost your excess weight. Visualize yourself walking into one of your favourite clothing stores. As you look at the clothes in your 'new', smaller size, select an outfit that you find attractive. Make sure it is one that will show off your figure. How about a swimsuit? Now go into the dressing room and try the outfit on. Come out and look at yourself in the mirror. You look terrific! Try to imagine what you would actually be feeling. What a sense of accomplishment! Look at your lean body. Feel the exhilaration and pride. Let yourself experience the excitement of the moment. The outfit really flatters your new shape.

It's important to visualize this scene as clearly and as vividly as you can. Use all of your senses. See, hear, feel, and touch what is happening. Use different items on your list each time. After your little mental trip into the future, you will feel a renewed strong sense of commitment and a much greater resolve.

Practice Makes Perfect

Planning ahead is an important part of dieting and motivation. In Chapter 15 I advised you to review your progress and plan ahead on a regular basis. As you look ahead from week to week, try to figure out what obstacles might get in your way. What might interfere with eating four meals every day or doing your Calorie Burners after meals? Are you worried about making it through a weekend visit from some old friends? Or perhaps you are going to have a particularly stressful time in your family or business life in the next week or two. Perhaps you are afraid you will be thrown off your eating and exercise schedule.

You must prepare yourself *before* these things happen. You must stay one step ahead of dietary menaces. You can use your imagination to get ready for these rough spots.

A day or two before the difficult situation is going to occur, put yourself through the following mental exercise. Close your eyes and imagine the difficult situation is happening *now*, not a day or two in the future, but *now*. Let's suppose that on Sunday evening you will be alone at home. The weather has been terrible and you have been a bit down in the dumps lately. You have been sticking to the diet very well, but you are worried about Sunday night. You realize that when you are alone, feeling restless and bored, you are more likely to break your diet.

On Saturday you should begin gathering your strengths about you. Close your eyes and imagine that Sunday evening has arrived. You visualize yourself at home in the kitchen. You feel a momentary craving to eat a favourite high-calorie food. Immediately, you take a deep breath and slowly let it out. Once again, you take a deep breath and then exhale slowly. You tell yourself to relax. You think back over the dinner you had three hours ago. The diet called for spaghetti tonight, and you really enjoyed it. You concentrate on how enjoyable the meal was and how full it made you feel. You tell yourself to relax. Gradually, you feel your hunger going away. You begin to relax, to breathe more regularly. The craving has passed. You feel physically and psychologically in control.

Now imagine you leave the kitchen and get involved in a favourite book, television show, or hobby. Perhaps you telephone a friend. You think to yourself, 'I really don't feel deprived at all. I'm going to relax and enjoy the evening. Besides, I'll be eating my metabo-meal in about an hour anyway.'

Then you visualize yourself an hour later, eating one of your favourite metabo-meals. Thirty minutes later you are on your exercise bicycle burning calories. You are satisfied and totally committed to your diet and exercise plan.

Going through this scene in your imagination, keeping a positive in-control feeling, builds confidence in your ability to stick with the programme. By repeating this visualization several times, you help yourself think through problems and solve them before they occur. You also brainwash yourself. By the time Sunday evening arrives, the real situation will seem easy, just like another mental practice session.

Use this technique whenever you foresee that your diet or exercise plan may be threatened. Use this preparation to plan ways to help yourself succeed. And keep your images positive. See yourself succeeding. Never even consider failure.

Excuses, Excuses, Excuses

From time to time we all use excuses to avoid exercise or to eat more calories than we should. It is human nature to give yourself an 'acceptable' reason for not sticking to your plan of action. What is even more frustrating is the fact that we all use the *very same* excuses over and over again. It is only later, after you have overeaten or missed your exercise, that you 'see through' the flimsy excuse.

You must be aware of excuses, identify them for what they are, and counterattack with a stronger argument.

Here are some typical excuses along with a counterattack for each. If you hear yourself making an excuse, immediately replace it with a more positive 'counterattack' thought.

Excuse No. 1: But I have tried other diets and failed. It is just impossible for me to lose weight.

Counterattack: The reason I failed before is because I went about it the wrong way. The Hilton Head Metabolism Diet is completely different. This is finally my chance to succeed, never to have to diet again.

Excuse No. 2: I have been just as faithful to the diet as my husband has, and he is losing faster than I am. I am getting discouraged.

Counterattack: Men are supposed to lose faster than women because of their higher metabolic rates. Besides, the reason I am on this programme is because my metabolism is sluggish. If I give it a chance, my metabolism will pick up, and I will be burning more calories than I ever have before.

Excuse No. 3: It is impossible to fit in all these meal and exercise times with a schedule like mine.

Counterattack: Nothing is impossible if I want it badly enough. I may have to do some creative time management, but *I can do it.*

Excuse No. 4: I don't have any willpower.

Counterattack: I don't need any more willpower than anyone else. Willpower is simply planning ahead and wanting to succeed. Besides, the Hilton Head Metabolism Diet is easy to follow, and I don't have to be a saint to stick to the rules.

Excuse No. 5: I am too nervy and upset right now. I will just have to get off the diet and get back on it later.

Counterattack: Being nervy and upset about things happening in my life should have nothing to do with dieting and exercise. Good nutrition and regular exercise help me cope with the stresses, strains, and emotional upsets of life. Being depressed or upset or angry is *not* a good reason to eat or skip exercise. What I should be doing is trying to solve the problem, finding a sympathetic friend who will lend an ear, or learning better skills to deal with emotional stress.

Excuse No. 6: I hate dieting. I always feel so deprived.

Counterattack: The Hilton Head Metabolism Diet is different. I really do not feel deprived. It is a positive approach. I feel that for the first time in my life I am doing the right thing to control my weight. I feel positive and satisfied with the diet.

Excuse No. 7: I am going on holiday for a week. I will just have to get back on the diet when I come home.

Counterattack: I *can* go on holiday at the same time. The Hilton Head Metabolism Diet fits easily into any schedule. In fact, it may be even easier on holiday because my time is my own.

Excuse No. 8: Everybody else at this party is eating and drinking whatever they want. It's not fair that I have to diet.

Counterattack: My diet is only temporary. And the faster I get my metabolism back to normal, the faster I will be able to eat like everyone else. If I give in now, it will only slow my progress and take my metabolism longer to get into shape.

Friendly Enemies

Your family and friends can have a tremendous effect on your motivation. They can encourage you and help you keep going. On the other hand, they can do or say things that have the reverse effect. If you have ever gone off a diet out of anger or spite, then you know exactly what I am talking about. There are four particularly damaging types of remarks you sometimes hear from family and friends.

CRITICAL REMARKS

Critical remarks about you or your diet can be quite discouraging. Ever hear such comments as 'Oh no, not another diet!' or (especially on the Hilton Head Metabolism Diet) 'Spaghetti!? I never heard of a diet that allows that. Are you sure you're not cheating?'

PESSIMISTIC REMARKS

Some people react negatively to just about everything, but especially to diets. They will try to discourage you by saying, 'No diet is permanent. You will just gain it all back,' or 'I know you will never last more than a few days.'

PERMISSIVE REMARKS

Some people feel sorry for you. In an attempt to be 'nice' they give you excuses to go off the diet (as if you didn't have enough of your own). They say, 'Go ahead. That ice cream won't hurt you,' or 'Don't worry. It doesn't matter if you don't exercise for a couple of days.' Sometimes these are overweight friends looking for company.

SUPERVISORY REMARKS

Probably the most infamous of all friendly enemies is what I call the *dietary supervisor*. This person tries to 'help' you by taking control of your diet. He or she assumes that since you have failed at diets before, you need someone to look after you. They say, 'Don't forget to do your exercise today' or 'Now let's make sure *this* diet works' or 'Now don't be eating anything you're not supposed to today.' These remarks only make you want to eat more, exercise less, and throw something (preferably something large and heavy) at your self-appointed supervisor.

The difficult part about dealing with these comments is that they usually come from those who care about you the most. Keep in mind that these people are trying to help you. They are not hostile, vindictive, or out to get you. They are just misguided. They simply do not understand dieting, and they may not understand you very well either. Just don't be overly sensitive to their comments. Remind yourself that their intentions are good, but that they just don't understand.

When these remarks occur often or when these comments make it more difficult for you to stick to the diet, you may have to let people know how they are affecting you. Don't be shy. Just tell them in a direct, straightforward manner that, even though they are trying to help, their remarks are having a negative effect. You must convince them that for you to succeed, *you* and you alone must be responsible for that success. You want their encouragement, of course, but not their criticism, advice, or supervision.

Also, ask family members *not* to:

- tease you about your diet,
- offer you foods you are not supposed to eat,
- repeatedly ask how many pounds you have lost,
- give you advice,
- remind you to stick to your diet,
- admonish or lecture you if you 'slip'.

Temporary Setbacks

What should you do if in spite of your best efforts you slip a bit? First, remember that you are human and subject to error from time to time. A slip does *not* mean you are a failure. It does *not* mean you don't have willpower. It simply means you are human, like everyone else. Second, do *not*, under any circumstances, allow yourself to feel guilty. Guilt will just make you feel worse and keep you from getting back on the straight and narrow.

Avoid such thoughts as 'Well, I have really blown it now. Maybe I'll get back on the programme next week.' Get back on the programme *immediately*. In fact, try not to think in terms of being *on* or *off* the diet. If you slip, consider it a slight deviation from the plan. You are only slightly off course. Do not act as if your ship has sunk.

Profit from your mistakes. If you missed your after-meal exercise today, figure out what went wrong. How could you have fitted your exercise in? Could you have arranged your schedule differently? Once you have figured this out, forget about your slip. Turn your mistake into a good lesson. Once it's over, forget it.

Never, ever compensate for a slip by missing a meal. Even if you eat a chocolate bar at 4:00 P.M., eat your dinner as planned. Remember, skipping meals is a very, very bad habit and especially bad for your metabolism. If you feel a need to undo your wrongdoing, exercise a little more that day or the next.

I believe you will find the Hilton Head Metabolism Diet so different and so challenging that slips will rarely occur. You will feel positive, and you will be making progress every day. You *can* do it. I want to make this the last diet of your life. I have faith in you. Just remember to have faith in yourself.

17

Being Realistic about Dieting

You don't have to become a hermit to stick to the Hilton Head Metabolism Diet. I want you to live your life exactly the way you do when you're not dieting. That means at restaurants and dinner parties, and on business trips and holidays. If you avoid these situations, you'll feel 'different' and deprived. You'll soon become bored and restless and feel sorry for yourself. And before you know it, there goes the diet. Besides, you must get used to dealing with every possible eating situation.

Watch Your Attitude

Forget about your past diets and past failures. Since the Hilton Head Metabolism Diet emphasizes calories burned up more than calories eaten, you can stay on the diet and live a normal life at the same time. You don't have to panic about eating out.

On other diets you may have had a tendency to get lax when not eating at home. Perhaps it was easy to give yourself an excuse for going off the diet. You may have thought, 'How can anyone diet at a dinner party? It's unheard of!'

I'm telling you it's not only possible, it's easy. Remember:

NO EATING SITUATION EXISTS
THAT YOU CANNOT HANDLE.

Don't be afraid or give up when you eat out. View the experience as a *challenge*. Accept the challenge and face it head on. The Hilton Head Metabolism Diet menus are such that they can easily be adapted to *any* situation.

Restaurants

The first rule in dealing successfully with restaurants is to plan ahead. Try to choose a restaurant with a varied menu. Ethnic restaurants are fine occasionally, but they make it much more difficult for you to stick to the diet.

It also helps to plan out the exact type of meal you will be ordering. This is a lot easier if you are familiar with the restaurant you're going to. The first step in this planning process is to look at my menus to determine what you're supposed to be having that day. If possible, plan to order exactly what I have prescribed. Slight variations of vegetables or fruits would certainly be allowed. Check my substitution lists in Chapter 19.

If you feel you'll have difficulty ordering the meal for that day, simply choose the corresponding meal from another day. For example, if while on the Low-cal menus you are going out to lunch on Tuesday, you might find the restaurant unable to serve you an egg on wholemeal bread. Then you could substitute Thursday's lunch, which calls for a tossed salad. This works out particularly well if the restaurant has a salad bar. Wednesday's tuna fish meal might be appropriate, except most restaurants carry oil-packed rather than water-packed tuna, which would add considerably to the calories. If you're not sure, ask whether the tuna was packed in oil or water.

Your biggest enemy at the salad bar is the salad dressing. Those dips of blue cheese, French, or Italian dressings contain as many calories by themselves as *two* of my Low-cal lunches. Either take your own diet dressing, or use vinegar and lemon. Oil has 100 calories per tablespoon – much too much for you unless you're in Reentry or Maintenance. Unfortunately, most restaurants do not routinely have diet salad dressing. Try to find the ones that do and take your business to them.

If you're going out to dinner, the easiest meals to order would be my Tuesday, Thursday, Saturday, or Sunday Low-cal dinners or my Wednesday, Thursday, Friday, or Saturday dinners on the Booster programme. These meals call for fish, chicken, beef, veal, lamb, prawns, or pasta. All of these are easy to obtain in just about any restaurant. If during the Low-cal programme, you're eating out at a steakhouse on Sunday evening, simply substitute Saturday's steak dinner for your pre-scribed Sunday spaghetti dinner. Eat your spaghetti on Saturday night. On the other hand, if you're at an Italian restaurant on Saturday night, substitute in the opposite direction. Eat your spaghetti, and enjoy the steak on Sunday night.

Here are some basic restaurant rules for you to keep in mind:

- Always make sure to order your fish grilled *without* butter.

- Don't be hesitant to ask about portion sizes – e.g. how many ounces is the steak? If you're supposed to have four or five ounces (that's *after* cooking), try *not* to end up with a ten-ounce steak on your plate. If you do, eat half and put the other half aside.

- If you're ordering steak, make sure you cut off all visible fat before eating it.

- If your menu calls for diet margarine on the

potato but the restaurant doesn't carry it, use half the amount of regular margarine.

- Make sure that no sauces are added to your entrée. You may have to give the waiter or waitress specific instructions about this.

- Make sure no salad dressing, croutons, or bacon bits are added to your salad.

- Order your vegetables plain, with no butter or sauces added.

- Remove the skin from your chicken before eating it.

- Order fresh fruit for dessert if it's available. If they only have tinned fruit, forget it. Tinned fruit is usually packed in sugary syrup. If they don't have fresh fruit and your menu calls for it, have extra fruit at home with your metabo-meal.

- Since salt is used freely in restaurant kitchens, be careful about adding extra salt when you're eating out. Just don't use the salt shaker. You may retain extra fluid, which will temporarily add weight.

- Ask questions of the waiter or waitress and be specific about exactly what you want.

- *You* are the customer; *you* are paying the bill, and it's their job to accommodate you.

If you end up at a speciality or ethnic restaurant, you can still order something that is low in calories. You may have difficulty sticking strictly to the menus I have outlined; try to abide by them with as few variations as possible.

Italian restaurants are adaptable to the diet, since they serve veal, chicken, and pasta dishes, all of which are acceptable on the diet. It's the cheeses, stuffings, sauces, and wine you must avoid. Veal Piccata (with lemon and wine sauce) is an excellent entrée and is only 350 calories.

While my wife, Gabrielle, was in the process of losing thirty pounds some time ago (pounds she has never gained back), we ate in a popular Italian restaurant in New York City. She first ordered a small salad with vinegar as the dressing. For her entrée she ordered a stuffed lamb chop, which was the closest menu item to the Hilton Head Metabolism Diet menu for that night. She ate the chop and left the stuffing. The lamb chop was accompanied by green beans, which she ordered without butter. The waiter was at first a bit taken aback by her apparent lack of appetite for the special 'dishes of the house', but, after a little explanation and joking back and forth, he was extremely accommodating. He could have done with losing a few pounds himself, and by the end of our dinner seemed quite in awe of her willpower.

Another excellent choice in an Italian restaurant is my Sunday spaghetti meal. Just make sure the tomato sauce is plain (no meat) and that you ask for a small portion. Remember, you can even have the Italian bread with the spaghetti dinner. Doesn't sound like being deprived, does it?

Chinese food can be okay if you're careful. If you have high blood pressure or retain fluid easily, watch out for the soy sauce and the monosodium glutamate (MSG). Generally speaking, Chinese food is low in calories. However, avoid egg rolls, dumplings, and spareribs. Stick to dishes that are boiled, steamed, or poached rather than stir-fried with oil. Avoid pork and sausage dishes. Chicken or prawn dishes are probably your best bets. I would suggest Chicken Subgum (chicken with vegetables), Egg Foo Yong, Sweet and Sour Prawns, or Chicken with Snow Peas. Avoid any dishes with nuts.

French restaurants are a particular challenge because of their penchant for sauces loaded with cream, butter, and eggs. Avoid these sauces while dieting, because the calories are deadly. A simply prepared grilled fish such as a striped bass is a good choice. Roast Chicken (*Poularde Rotie*), medallions of beef (*Medallions de Filet de Boeuf*), or peppered filet mignon (*Filet Mignon au Poivre Flambé*) are excellent meals for your diet. The entrée can be accompanied by a vegetable (no sauce, please) and a potato (baked, not French fried). For dessert you can have fresh fruit (plain, with no topping), which is readily available in most French restaurants.

Dinner Parties

You must also be able to contend with dinners at the homes of friends or business associates. In these situations your choices are more limited than in restaurants, but don't worry, you can handle it. Small dinners with intimate friends are often easier, since most friends will know you're dieting and try to accommodate you. Maybe you'll be really lucky, and your friends will join you on the Hilton Head Metabolism Diet. One of my patients arrived at a friend's dinner party and, to her delight and relief, was served my Poussin dinner from the Booster week menu, exactly as I described it. It seemed that the hostess had just begun the Hilton Head Metabolism Diet two weeks earlier and was determined to stick to my plan in spite of her dinner party. Everyone enjoyed the meal and no one, except my patient, knew they had just enjoyed a low-calorie diet meal.

Don't panic if the dinner party starts with cocktails and hors d'oeuvres. Arrive a little late and quickly get yourself a soda water or Perrier with lime or lemon. Position yourself as far away from the hors d'oeuvres as possible, and get involved in an interesting conversation. As you watch others eating and drinking, try to feel a little superior to them. *You* are changing your metabolism while they continue to suppress theirs. Go ahead. It's okay to feel snobbish. After all, you've found the secret to dieting success once and for all.

If the dinner party is like most I've attended, be prepared to eat later than usual. To prepare for this, I suggest you have your metabo-meal in the late afternoon, even if you typically have it later, after dinner. You might also plan to eat lunch later that day, say around 1:30 P.M., then not have your metabo-meal until 5:30 P.M. Also, make sure you get your after-meal exercises in early that day. You may not eat dinner until 9:00 P.M. or 9:30 P.M., and you'll probably sit around socializing afterwards. By the time you arrive home, it's doubtful if you'll exercise. So plan your thermal walks or other energy-burning exercises after breakfast and lunch.

If the dinner is served buffet style, you'll at least be able to pick and choose what you want. If a salad is available, give yourself a generous portion. Next, choose the vegetable, unless it's covered in butter or a sauce. Potatoes, of course, are fine. If the main dish is simply too fattening, either take just a small amount or leave it altogether. Remember, you don't have to eat everything that's available.

If there's no buffet and you're simply served a prepared meal, do the best you can. Chicken, fish, beef, pasta, vegetables, potatoes, and fruit are your basic foods. Eat those if they're served. Avoid casseroles or dishes with sauces. Leave foods you should not have. After all, losing weight and changing your metabolism are serious matters. It's a little like treating yourself for a disease – the disease of *metabolic suppression*. So don't take it lightly. If you don't stick to the diet as closely as possible day after day, you'll simply be slowing your progress. I'm sure you don't want your weight loss to take any longer than is necessary.

If the host and hostess are close friends or relatives, you may want to let them know about your diet when you accept the invitation. In most cases I'm sure they'll try to give you what you need.

Once you arrive at the dinner party, you must be able to refuse offers of certain foods that are definitely off-limits. Say, 'no' to the wine and say 'no' to dessert, unless it's fresh fruit, of course. You're not going to hurt anyone's feelings. Whether you realize it or not, most of your friends couldn't care less about what you eat. And no one is going to tempt you, especially if they know you're on the Hilton Head Metabolism Diet. Be gracious but firm. Say, 'No, thank you. I don't care for dessert, but I would like a cup of that great coffee of yours. By the way, Flo, that meal was delicious.'

There's one more thing. Many people who are overweight get a little paranoid when it comes to eating in public. They feel as if everyone is watching to see what they are or are not eating. That's nonsense. No one is looking at you. They're too busy paying attention to their own food. If they do notice you, they'll probably be impressed and want to know all about your new diet.

One final word about dinner parties: I have found that increasing your exercise the day before, the day of, and the day after the party has a tremendous impact on your commitment and resolve. Try to exercise after *three* meals each day instead of only two. That way, should you eat a few extra calories, they'll be burned off quickly and won't affect your progress.

Travelling for Business or Pleasure

Whether you're on a short holiday or a business trip, you can still follow the Hilton Head Metabolism Diet.

The first problem arises during the course of travel by plane or car. If you're flying to your destination, find out in advance if a meal will be served on the aircraft. If so, call and arrange for a special meal. This is a routine procedure; the airlines are used to it. While they won't prepare different individual menus, they will serve a low-calorie meal. Ask for either the low-calorie meal, the diabetic meal, or the low-sodium meal. All of these are nutritionally well balanced and low in calories. In fact, these meals are always more appetizing and attractively served than the regular meal everyone else is getting. Be sure to order your special food ahead of time, when you make your reservation, or they probably won't be able to accommodate you.

If your flight is just a short hop or a series of short hops, try to arrange your meals so you're eating before you leave and upon your arrival. If you end up eating in an airport, avoid the little snack and hot dog stands; take the time to go to the large, more varied cafeteria-style restaurants most airports have. If you're eating lunch, choose a salad or fruit platter. For dinner, chicken is standard cafeteria fare and a good choice, unless it's fried. If nothing looks appropriate, have a salad or fruit platter for dinner, then make up the calories at your metabo-meal.

If you're really pressed for time, buy a piece of fruit and eat it as your metabo-meal. Then eat your lunch or dinner when you have the opportunity. You might even bring fruit with you from home, so you'll be prepared.

And don't just sit around the airport. Have your meal, whether large or small, wait twenty minutes, and get walking. Airports can be a great place to walk. Just keep yourself moving while you're waiting for the plane. Most passengers sit or stand for an hour or more, feeling bored and wasting time. You can be stirring up your metabolism, taking advantage of the extra time to burn more calories. There's a regular traveller in the Atlanta airport who takes along his jogging clothes, changes in the rest room, and runs while waiting for his next connection.

If you're travelling by car, plan your trip carefully. Try to allow enough time for meals. If you're rushed to get where you're going, you won't take the time to eat properly. Take a picnic meal with you if you are in a big hurry. Most of my meals can be prepared ahead of time and taken along in the car. If you'll be eating at a roadside restaurant, avoid the fast food places. Try to find a family restaurant that could serve you at least an approximation of your diet meals. It might take a little more time, but isn't your weight problem worth it? If a fast food restaurant is all that's available, choose one with a salad bar.

When you're taking a meal with you in the car, make sure you take *only* that meal. Some families get into the habit of loading the car with snack foods, even if the destination is only two or three hours away. This sets a bad precedent for all concerned. And don't eat your diet meal whenever you feel hungry. Set a definite meal time, stop the car, and take time to eat. If you're near a park or highway rest area, you may even be able to take a twenty-minute walk. This would allow you to stretch and also serve as your after-meal Calorie Burner.

Once you arrive at your destination, follow my menu plan whether you're preparing your own meals or eating out in restaurants. If, for example, you're staying with friends for the weekend, let them know about your diet ahead of time. They don't have to change their meal plans completely, but if they're friends, they'll certainly want to help you. Also, make certain you continue with the exercise plan. This is especially important when you are away from home and your routine is disrupted. Holidays, Bank Holiday weekends, and business trips are *not* an excuse for straying from the Hilton Head Metabolism Diet. You'll find staying with it a lot easier than you might think.

Business and Social Meals

In the course of dieting, you may be exposed to a business lunch or dinner or a club luncheon. I'm talking about those already prepared meals where everyone gets the same thing. Creamed chicken is definitely not on the diet. You basically have three choices on these occasions.

First, you could eat before or after the meal and just enjoy the meeting or the company of others without eating the prepared meal. Second, you could eat the salad and fruit, if available, as your metabo-meal and eat again later. Third, you could try to get by with the meal if it happens to be steak, plain chicken, or roast beef. Just pick and choose. Eat the salad, the entrée, and the vegetable; skip the dessert.

18

Preventing Metabolic Suppression in Children

I've had so many patients tell me, 'If I'd only known about your metabolism teachings when I was young, I could have kept myself slim.' If a person starts working on his metabolism when he's young, he'll be able to control his weight for the rest of his life. The best time to begin, of course, is during childhood.

If you are fat, you should be especially concerned about your children. In Chapter 2, I told you that a child with one overweight parent stands a 40 per cent greater chance of being overweight than if neither parent is overweight. If both parents are fat, the risk goes up to 80 per cent. So you should take immediate steps to protect your children from the problem, even if they are slim. You'll be preventing a future weight problem by tuning your child's metabolic engine and establishing habits that will keep that engine tuned for ever. It's a bit like inoculating him or her against measles or smallpox.

If any of your children are already overweight, get them started tomorrow. If you're waiting for the baby fat to disappear, you may have a *very* long wait. Fat children grow up to be fat adults.

Fat's Not Fun

Being fat can result in serious medical problems for children, just as it can in adults. Overweight children suffer even more, psychologically. They often feel inferior and 'different'. Other children make matters worse by calling them 'Fatso', 'Fatty', or other derogatory names. Fat children can react by becoming shy and withdrawn or by developing unruly behaviour problems. They become the class bully or the class clown, demanding attention through silly, immature actions.

Children develop attitudes and stereotypes about fat people very early in life. Simply because they are fat, overweight children are thought to be unattractive, lazy, sloppy, gluttonous, and unintelligent. These judgements are made solely on the basis of appearance and are extremely unfair. Adults as well as children are guilty of passing along these stereotypes. Even doctors are not immune – studies show that doctors have a more negative emotional reaction to fat children than to even severely deformed youngsters.

Fat children avoid physical activities and athletics because they have more difficulty moving their bodies than other children. They are often slower and weaker than other kids. They dread physical education classes for fear of embarrassment and failure. The lack of exercise makes their weight problem worse. They never develop the athletic skills needed to make sports fun. This can also lead to a lifelong dislike for exercise of any type. Chronic inactivity compounds the weight problem and practically ensures that it will become a permanent condition.

These patterns must be stopped early in life before they cause excessive metabolic damage. I wish every parent could know about metabolic suppression and prevent it in their children before it has a chance to get a foothold.

Don't despair if your child is overweight or has the heredity to be overweight. You can change your child's habits, and you can stir up his or her metabolism. Your child will never have to go on one unsuccessful diet after another, as you may have done. Now you have the knowledge to keep him or her trim and slim for ever.

Preventing Overweight

An increasing number of parents are worried about their children's health. They want to teach their children proper eating habits early in life so they grow up to be healthy adults. The only trouble is that most parents don't know how to go about it. Their intentions are good, but they don't know exactly what to teach. Other parents try to force good eating habits on their children and then wonder why the children rebel by eating sweets and junk foods.

I'm going to show you specifically what to do to prevent your child from getting fat in childhood or as an adult. Now's your chance to exert influence, before he or she gets to be a fat adult. Can you imagine how your life might have been different if my book had been available to your parents? You might have learned habits as a child that would have increased your metabolism. Then you never would have had a weight problem.

If your child is of average weight, and you want to protect him/her from ever being fat, you only have to follow a few simple suggestions.

FOUR MEALS EVERY DAY

You should get everybody in the family to eat four meals every day instead of three. Your children can have their fourth meal as a snack after school or later in the evening. Make sure they eat all four meals, including breakfast. Discourage other eating. Four meals will discourage snacking. Talk to your family about the change in the number of meals. Discuss how four meals helps to stimulate metabolism through the thermic effect. I find that most children are fascinated by my metabolism ideas.

CARBOHYDRATES FOR EVERYONE

Children should be taught about the best nutritional balance for daily eating. They will learn best by example, by your stimulating their interest in what they are learning. You must make it fun. Avoid lecturing or dictating. Your lectures will be greeted by deaf ears; your decrees will become challenges to do the opposite. I know of several parents who tell their children, 'Sweets and chocolate are bad for you. You must never, ever eat chocolate or sweets.' These are the same children who at school trade their peanut butter and wholemeal bread sandwiches for sweets and chocolate cake.

You cannot dictate nutritional rules to children. They don't understand them, especially when all their friends are eating whatever they please. You must avoid such absolutes as *never*. The rule of never eating anything sweet is absurd. There is nothing wrong with eating sweets occasionally. The problem arises when you eat too many of them, too often. The advice to give your child should be, 'Eat *fewer* sweets.'

You should explain why certain foods are better than others. Explain the types of foods that contain carbohydrates, protein, and fat. (See Chapter 4.) Get your children interested in food and nutrition. Make it interesting. Discuss food, calories, and metabolism casually at mealtime or any time you have the opportunity. Share this information with your child, don't thrust it on her. Say, 'Peggy, I learned something interesting about potatoes today,' rather than 'Peggy, it's about time you learned something about nutrition. Now, sit down here, and I'm going to teach you a few things.' And *never* say, 'Peggy, your eating habits are awful. From now on we're going to have different rules about food.'

Try to interest your children in looking at the lists of ingredients in packaged foods. Make a game out of it. Take any packaged food from your kitchen – let's say, peanut butter. See who in the family can correctly guess the most ingredients. When you serve meals, point out to the children that the salad, vegetable, potato, and fruit are carbohydrate foods, that at least half of your diet should contain these nutrients. Next, discuss the chicken, fish, or beef as protein foods and how only about 20 per cent of your daily food intake should be protein. Then describe the fats in the meat, salad dressing, or margarine.

Teach your children to limit their intake of salt. Change the salt in your shaker to one of the lighter salt products that are half sodium and half potassium. Don't add as much salt when cooking. If your child is doing a school project, encourage him to choose a topic related to nutrition, metabolism, dieting, or exercise.

EXERCISE AND PLENTY OF IT

If your child is already physically active, you're lucky. He or she is burning calories and enjoying it, too. Now, I'm not just talking about fidgety activity or hyperactivity. I'm referring to a genuine interest in games, sports, and physical movement – the type of interest that is healthy and can be sustained over a lifetime.

If your child is only moderately active or not active at all, you must start encouraging more activity. You must first and foremost be a good example. Your child must see *you* walking, cycling, playing tennis, swimming, or playing badminton. I don't just mean sports activities either. Your child must learn to value exercise for the sake of exercise. He or she must learn the rule that you don't develop fitness by playing sports, you develop fitness to enable you to play sports.

When done consistently, walking and cycling are probably the best all-around physical activities for helping to prevent weight problems. If, while they're young, you take your children for frequent walks, they'll be learning a valuable habit. As they get older, talk to them about metabolism and exercise. When you walk together or cycle together after meals, tell them about the connection between the thermic effect of meals and the results of exercising thirty minutes after meals. Teach them that metabolism is related to muscle tissue – the more muscle, the higher the metabolic rate. Exercise develops muscle and burns a lot of calories.

Above all, make exercise fun. Encourage, but don't push. Exercise in the form of walking, family badminton, tennis, swimming, or just playing catch can be a great time for everyone. Just make sure these activities occur frequently, not just once or twice a year on family holidays. Occasional exercise at weekends doesn't count either. You want your child to like being physically active almost every day.

Try to interest your children in physical games and athletics. When they're young, just make sure they learn the rules and participate. Don't pressure and criticize. Ask yourself, 'What is my goal?' The answer: to develop a real interest in activity in your child, not to make him the best tennis or football player in the world. Once he starts developing a real interest in several types of physical activity, if he shows the ability, then encourage him to excel in one or two sports. These activities are going to help your child control his weight in later years. But emphasize a longlasting activity level. If your son is later in the business world, how often is he going to be playing football?

Encourage your child to build more physical activitiy into everyday routines. Don't drive him or her every-where. Suggest walking or riding a bicycle to a friend's house, if it's not too far. Be a good example. When you drive to the shopping centre or grocery store together, park in the far corner of the car park. Point out what you're doing and how easy it is to increase physical activity in everyday life. If your child is young, make a game of coming up with new ways in which you both can be more active.

The Hilton Head Metabolism Diet
for Fat Children

If your child is already overweight, start him on the Hilton Head Metabolism Diet. Better yet, go on it together. If everyone in the family needs to lose a few pounds, make it a family project. It's a lot easier when more than one person in the household is dieting.

Before you begin, consult your family doctor, who will be familiar with your child's health and weight history and able to advise on any special dietary precautions. Your doctor can also provide supervision and answer any specific medical questions you might have.

Children need more calories than adults even when dieting. They can lose weight as well or even better than adults, on more calories. Because of age and a short or non-existent history of fad dieting, they will have only a slight problem with metabolic suppression. The metabolic suppression they have is most likely due to excess body fat, a limited amount of lean body mass, and too little exercise.

Because of nutritional requirements for proper growth and development, I would not recommend that children under eighteen years of age be put on anything less than a 1000-calorie diet. Therefore, I do not recommend the use of my Low-cal menus for children and young teenagers. Instead, they should be put on my Booster meals as their basic diet. These meals will provide them with adequate calories and sufficient proteins, carbohydrates, and fats for their growing bodies. After two weeks of Booster, they should be switched to one week of Reentry, then go back to Booster again. Just as the adult menus call for two weeks of Low-cal interspersed with one week of Booster, children require two weeks of Booster followed by one week of Reentry.

When the child is within two pounds of his or her goal, keep him or her on the Reentry menus until the ideal weight is reached. Then let him/her go back to normal eating again, only try to keep the nutritional balance within the 20 per cent protein-55 per cent carbohydrate-25 per cent fat range.

During the diet, serve your child four meals every day. No other eating should be allowed. The metabo-meal would make a nice after-school snack. And my Booster metabo-meals include such foods as popcorn, bagels, and fresh fruit, which most children enjoy. Enough sandwiches are included in these menus to make school lunches easy.

If your child normally eats lunch at the school cafeteria, it would be better for him or her to take a packed lunch while dieting. Unless the school cafeteria is very special, or unless the school has a dietician who can help, choosing the appropriate lunch at school will be difficult and confusing for your child. However, eventually he or she must learn to make these choices.

Discuss the school lunch menu with your child each day. Decide together what might be a good low-calorie lunch. Make sure it includes mostly food items that he or she likes. Every once in a while let your child choose a lunch in the cafeteria instead of taking it from home. After school, go over the choice made. Don't act like a detective checking up on proper behaviour. Let your child get the feeling of being in charge of his or her diet – you are only an assistant. Make sure your dieting talks are two-way discussions, not one-sided lectures.

Exercise and the Fat Child

Your overweight child must do my Calorie Burners after two meals every day. If he or she is not yet in school, choose any two meals – probably after breakfast and lunch or after lunch and a late afternoon metabo-meal would be best. A walk, bike ride, or any sustained physical activity is great. Remember, wait thirty minutes *after* the meal, and then encourage exercise for twenty minutes. You will have to exercise with your child at first. Games that involve physical activity are good. Even a vigorous game of hide-and-seek, if he or she is actively looking for you most of the time, would be a great after-meal Calorie Burner.

If your child is older and in school, exercise after the late afternoon metabo-meal and dinner would be the most practical. The after-dinner Calorie Burner could be a family activity. In spring and summer months when the weather is nice, the whole family could go out for a walk twenty minutes after dinner. This will not only give your child needed exercise, but also give the family a nice 'togetherness' time. It will show your child that physical activity is important to you and everyone else in the family. Before long your child will look forward to this family activity time.

Make sure the atmosphere is pleasant during these walks. Focus your attention on the children. Listen to them. Ask them questions. Make it *their* time. Make them feel that the exercise time is fun time and not drudgery. Be positive and have fun yourself. Use the time to enjoy your children and relax.

If the weather is bad, if it's dark, or if your neighbourhood is not safe for walking, schedule family activity indoors. Children of all ages love rebounders or bouncers, those minitrampolines I discussed in Chapter 12. Have family games to see who can bounce the longest, or see who can come up with new exercise variations. If you have an exercise bicycle, see how many miles each family member can go in twenty minutes. Because of the time factor, one family member needs to be on the exercycle while another is on the rebounder. The third can be dancing and jumping around in time to music. The next night everyone can switch to a new activity. Use your imagination to come up with new exercises.

Praise your child frequently for progress made. Don't expect major changes right away. Look for small improvements in exercise patterns first. Don't expect him or her to be thrilled by the new programme. Your child will gradually get used to it and, with your encouragement and attention, learn to enjoy it (hopefully, for the rest of his life).

What to Do about a Chubby Baby

If your child is less than one year of age and a bit on the chubby side, you can get him or her started on the metabolism programme early. You don't have to put him or her on a diet. You just have to follow several simple rules.

CONSULT YOUR DOCTOR

If you are worried about your baby's weight, the first person to consult is your family doctor. Let him guide you and supervise any plan of action. Your baby needs certain basic nutrients, so your doctor's guidance is absolutely necessary.

DON'T OVERFEED

Feed your baby according to whatever schedule your doctor suggests. Breast milk and infant formula milk are the healthiest, with mother's breast milk less likely to contribute to overweight. Infants do not need cow's milk.

Most paediatricians recommend that solid foods not be added to the diet until four to six months of age. Solids should be added gradually at that point. Do not overfeed. If your baby seems full and content after eating half a jar of baby food, don't force him or her to eat the rest. Let your baby be the judge of how full he or she is. Never add sugar to solid foods to get your baby to eat them. Remember, you're trying to establish healthy habits. Natural juices are fine, but make sure you read the list of ingredients in any food you're feeding the baby.

And remember, your baby will gain three times as much weight in the first year of life as in the second. This is perfectly natural. Just realize that appetite will diminish in the second year, and don't be alarmed by that.

BE CAREFUL ABOUT SWEETS

You don't have to eliminate sweets completely as your infant gets older. As I mentioned before, strict limitations can often backfire on you. You must definitely avoid using chocolate, ice cream, biscuits, or other sweets as special treats or rewards. Many adults have fond memories of special outings with a parent to the local sweetshop or ice cream parlour – it was a special time of togetherness. But this is a definite 'no-no'. The special times can just as easily be walks in the woods or a game of catch. Avoid sweets as a reward. Also avoid giving sweets or snacks when your child is upset. You might momentarily be cheering him or her up, but you're teaching a very bad habit. As an adult, he or she may head straight for the refrigerator whenever tense, depressed, or angry. Is that really what you want to teach? Talk to your child, encouraging expression of feelings. Take your child for a walk to lift his or her spirits; don't feed him/her. It's almost like giving a two-year-old a tranquillizer every time he gets upset. That teaches him to abuse food, the way others too easily learn to abuse drugs.

ENCOURAGE ACTIVITY

Probably the most important thing you can do for a chubby baby is to encourage physical activity. As he or she begins to move around and crawl, encourage use of new skills. If he or she wants to crawl across the room to get a toy, fine. Encourage movement. Don't you fetch the toy; don't let a big sister or brother get it for the child. Look for opportunities to make your baby move his or her body. Buy toys that help keep the child active – toys that require manipulation. Educational puzzles and games are fine, but many of them stimulate only the mind. When you are bathing your baby, encourage arm and leg movements in the water. You might even sign up for a swimming class that teaches infants to swim with the mother's assistance. See if there's one in your community.

19

Substitutions

To provide a little more flexibility on the diet, I'm giving you a list of substitutes for the fruits, vegetables, and protein foods on my menus. Keep in mind that the closer you stick to my menu plans, the better you'll do – and the faster you'll lose weight. But I do realize that some vegetables and fruits are easier to buy at certain times of the year. Since I strongly advise fresh fruits and vegetables, you'll need to know about substitutions as the seasons vary. I also realize that you may have allergies or strong likes or dislikes you want to take into account.

Fruit

My menus often call for fruit, especially at breakfast. You can substitute any of the following fruits for one another in the same proportion. One half piece of any of the following is approximately equal in calories.

Apple	Pear
Banana	Orange
Grapefruit	Nectarine
Tangerine	

Other fruits vary in their calorie content. To make substitutions easy for you, the following list gives you the portions of different fruits that are equal to a half section of any of the above fruits. You can substitute any of these fruits for one another or for the above list, as long as you use the portion indicated.

Apricots	2 whole
Blackberries	50g (2oz)
Blackcurrants	50g (2oz)
Raspberries	50g (2oz)
Strawberries	100g (4oz)
Fig	1 whole
Grapes	75g (3oz)
Mango	1 whole
Cantaloupe	¼
Honeydew	⅛
Watermelon	100g (4oz)
Papaya	¾
Peach	1 whole
Persimmon	1 whole
Pineapple	60g (2½oz)
Plums	2 whole
Prunes	2 whole
Raisins	1½ tablespoons

Vegetables

The following are what I call the *Group I* vegetables: 100g (4oz) of any of these can be substituted for any other. So, if my menu calls for green beans or asparagus, you can substitute any of the following, as long as it's the same portion.

Asparagus	Okra
Green beans	Marrow
Broccoli	Carrots
Brussels sprouts	Rhubarb
Cauliflower	Tomatoes
Cabbage	Turnips
Aubergine	Kale
Collard greens	Turnip greens
Spring greens	Courgettes
Spinach	Beetroot

The following are my *Group II* vegetables. These contain about three times as many calories as the Group I vegetables. They each can be substituted for one another, but *never* substitute a Group I vegetable with a Group II vegetable. You can substitute in the other direction. If your menu calls for corn on the cob, you can substitute 12oz (350g) of a Group I vegetable. (You can have three times as much of a Group I vegetable.)

Corn	Peas
Corn on the cob	Parsnips
Broad beans	

Protein Foods

Because of strong likes or dislikes or allergies, you may have to substitute one protein food for another. I suggest you avoid any substitutions of this type unless you have a definite allergy or unless you get physically ill eating certain foods. Make sure you follow my portions when you substitute, so you keep the calories the same.

Beef	25g (1oz)
Lamb	25g (1oz)
Veal	25g (1oz)
Chicken (without skin)	25g (1oz)
Turkey (without skin)	25g (1oz)
Poussin (without skin)	25g (1oz)
Fish	40g (1½oz)
Cottage cheese	50g (2oz)
Egg	1 whole (small)

Remember, however, certain foods – beef, for example – contain more fat, and by substituting you will be throwing off the nutritional balance of the diet.

Likes, Dislikes, and Allergies

Avoid changes in my basic menu plans at all costs. If you dislike vegetables, learn to like them. Before you resist a food, give yourself a fighting chance. Try just a little of foods that are not your favourites. I've included such a variety of normal, everyday foods that almost everybody can stick to the Hilton Head Metabolism Diet easily.

Once you start limiting what you can and cannot eat and making exceptions and substitutions, you've changed the diet. Then you're not on the Hilton Head Metabolism

Diet, you're on your own diet. So then when it doesn't work, don't blame the Hilton Head Metabolism Diet.

If you really have food allergies, you might want to go over the diet with your doctor. Let him or her guide and supervise any substitutions you may need.

20

Hilton Head
Metabolism Diet Recipes

If you are going to be on the Hilton Head Metabolism Diet for more than two weeks, these recipes will provide a little variety. Just make sure you continue to follow my menu plans.

The recipes have been planned so you can substitute a chicken recipe for chicken on the menu plans, fish for fish, pasta for pasta, and so on. In some cases I have adjusted the portion of chicken, fish, beef, or pasta slightly to compensate for some of the extra calories in the recipe. In this way you can freely substitute recipes for the equivalent dishes on my menu plans.

Chicken, Fish, and Beef

LADY DAPHNE'S CHICKEN

2 medium chicken breasts (about 150g (5oz) meat)
¼ teaspoon dried rosemary
1 tablespoon natural yoghurt

Remove skin from chicken and place chicken in ungreased baking pan. Bake for 30 minutes at 180°C (350°F) Gas 4. Remove from oven and cover with yoghurt. Sprinkle with rosemary leaves. Return to oven for 15 minutes then serve.

Serves 1

MEXICAN CHICKEN

1 medium tomato (fresh)
1 teaspoon lemon juice
½ teaspoon prepared mustard
4 tablespoons low-fat natural yoghurt
½ teaspoon sugar substitute
1 teaspoon dried parsley
1 teaspoon chilli powder
4 medium chicken breasts

Mix tomato, lemon juice, mustard, yoghurt, sugar substitute, parsley, and chilli powder in blender. Chill in refrigerator for one hour. Skin chicken and bake for 25 minutes at 180°C (350°F) Gas 4. Remove from oven and pour chilled sauce over chicken. Return to oven and bake for 20 minutes at 150°C (300°F) Gas 2.

Serves 4

SLIM CHICKEN CORDON BLEU

1 very thin slice bacon, rinds removed
4 chicken breasts (boneless and skinless)
50g (2oz) sliced or grated mozzarella cheese

Turn oven to 190°C (375°F) Gas 5. Place chicken pieces flat and side by side in a shallow baking pan. Place 8g (¼oz) cheese and half the slice of bacon on two of the breasts. Place a remaining breast on top of each of these. Bake at 190°C (375°F) Gas 5 for 35 minutes. Remove from oven, and place equal portions of the remaining cheese over each portion of chicken. Return to oven and cook for an additional 5 minutes.

Serves 2

QUICKY CHICKY BLUE

  150g (5oz) baked chicken
  1 tablespoon diet blue cheese salad dressing
  1 tablespoon chopped fresh parsley

Bake skinned chicken at 180°C (350°F) Gas 4 for 30 minutes. Remove from oven and top with salad dressing. Sprinkle with parsley. Add fresh ground pepper to taste. Wrap tightly in aluminium foil and return to oven for 15 to 20 minutes.

Serves 1

COQ AU VIN

  150g (5oz) baked chicken
  1 teaspoon fresh tarragon leaves
  50ml (2 fl oz) dry white wine

Place skinned chicken in baking dish. Sprinkle with tarragon leaves. Add wine. Cover with dish top or aluminium foil, and bake for one hour at 180°C (350°F) Gas 4.

Serves 1

CHICKEN STOCK

The next three dishes call for chicken stock. Here's the recipe.

  1 chicken carcass
  3½ litres (6 pints) water

Place carcass in water. Boil until liquid is reduced by half. Remove chicken and put stock in refrigerator overnight. When chilled, skim all fat from the top. Dispose of fat and use remaining stock for recipes.

JAMAICAN CHICKEN

  3 pineapple slices (water-packed)
  3 medium chicken breasts, skinned and boned
  ½ teaspoon instant coffee granules
  50ml (2 fl oz) chicken stock
  100ml (4 fl oz) low-fat natural yoghurt

Place pineapple slices in ungreased baking pan. Place a chicken breast on top of each. Dissolve coffee in boiling chicken stock. Stir in yoghurt. Pour mixture over chicken and bake at 190°C (375°F) Gas 5 for 40 minutes.

Serves 3

GABRIELLE'S CHICKEN A LA KING

  3 tablespoons diet margarine
  3 tablespoons flour
  350ml (12 fl oz) chicken stock
  275g (10oz) cooked chicken, chopped
  100g (4oz) chopped mushrooms
  100g (4oz) chopped pimento
  ¼ medium green pepper, chopped
  1½ tablespoons chopped onions

Melt margarine in large pan. Slowly blend in flour. Add chicken stock. Stir in all remaining ingredients. Cook over low heat for 10 minutes. For each serving allow 150g (5oz) over 1 slice diet bread or 60g (2½oz) cooked rice. (Omit potato from menu plan when using this recipe.)

Serves 4

CHICKEN (TURKEY) HASH

350ml (12 fl oz) chicken (turkey) stock
450g (1lb) cooked chicken (turkey), diced
2 small onions, chopped
3 celery stalks, chopped
2 medium green peppers, chopped
½ teaspoon dried thyme

To prepared stock in pot, add diced chicken (turkey) and all other ingredients. Cook on high heat for 5 minutes. Reduce to low heat and cook for 40 minutes. Measure out 150g (5oz) per person.

Serves 4

FISH DILL

700g (1½lb) fish of your choice (plaice, cod, coley)
50g (2oz) low-fat natural yoghurt
1½ teaspoons prepared horseradish
1 teaspoon dry mustard
½ teaspoon dill weed

Grill or bake fish according to taste. (As a general guideline, bake fish fillets at 190°C (375°F) Gas 5 for 20 to 25 minutes. Grill for 6 to 10 minutes, depending on thickness.) While fish is cooking, mix all other ingredients together in a small saucepan. Cook over low heat for 5 to 8 minutes, stirring occasionally. Pour sauce over cooked fish and serve.

Serves 4

FISH CREOLE

2 medium tomatoes, chopped
1 clove garlic, crushed
100g (4oz) chopped green peppers
100g (4oz) chopped onions
1 bay leaf (optional)
700g (1½lb) fish of your choice (plaice, cod, coley)

Mix tomatoes, garlic, peppers, onions, and bay leaf in small saucepan, and cook at low heat until tender. Pour over fish prior to baking or grilling. Either bake at 190°C (375°F) Gas 5 for 20 to 25 minutes, or grill for 6 to 10 minutes, depending on thickness.

Serves 4

PRAWN CURRY

2 tablespoons diet margarine
1 celery stalk, finely chopped
¼ apple, finely chopped
¼ small onion, finely chopped
50ml (2 fl oz) water
1½ teaspoons curry powder (1 tablespoon if you prefer a spicier dish)
100g (4oz) cottage cheese
1 tablespoon skimmed milk
350g (12oz) peeled prawns
pepper to taste

Melt margarine in large frying pan. Add celery, apple, and onion. Sauté. Add water and curry powder, and cook until most of the liquid has evaporated. While mixture is cooking, whip cottage cheese and skimmed milk in blender for 2 minutes. Add this cheese-milk mixture to the frying pan. Stir in prawns and add pepper to taste. Serve over 60g (2½oz) cooked rice.

Serves 2

MINCED BEEF STROGANOFF

450g (1lb) lean minced beef
100g (4oz) chopped onions
1 clove garlic, crushed
100g (4oz) chopped mushrooms
pepper to taste
1 tablespoon tomato purée
175ml (6 fl oz) warm water
2 tablespoons cooking sherry
225ml (8 fl oz) low-fat natural yoghurt

Brown beef in frying pan with onions and garlic. When beef is brown, add mushrooms and pepper. Stir in tomato purée and water. Cook over high heat for 5 minutes, stirring occasionally. Lower heat and add yoghurt and sherry to pan. Cook over low heat for 10 minutes. Serve over 50g (2oz) cooked egg noodles.

Serves 4

ALBERT'S MEAT LOAF

450g (1lb) lean minced beef
1 small onion, finely chopped
1 egg white
½ green pepper, finely chopped
2 celery stalks, finely chopped
1 teaspoon garlic powder

¼ teaspoon Tabasco sauce
¼ teaspoon dried sweet basil
¼ teaspoon dried oregano

Mix all ingredients thoroughly in a mixing bowl. Form into a loaf shape. Place in baking tin, and bake for 60 minutes at 170°C (325°F) Gas 3.

Serves 4

HERBAL HAMBURGER

175g (6oz) lean minced beef
1 pinch dried marjoram
1 pinch dried thyme
1 tablespoon dry red wine

Mix all ingredients together in a bowl. Form into patty. Grill for 5 to 8 minutes on each side.

Serves 1

TED'S VEAL PICCATA

450g (1lb) thinly sliced veal
pepper to taste
flour
4 tablespoons diet margarine
2 lemons
2 tablespoons chopped fresh parsley

Season veal to taste, then dust veal slices lightly with flour. Heat 2 tablespoons margarine in medium frying pan over medium to high heat. Add veal slices and brown for 2 to 3 minutes on each side. Remove veal and place on warm serving dish. Remove frying pan from heat and add juice of lemons, parsley, and remaining 2 tablespoons margarine. Stir thoroughly. Pour mixture over veal slices and serve.

Serves 3

PRAWNS WITH COCKTAIL SAUCE

450ml (¾ pint) water
2 medium tomatoes
15 drops Tabasco sauce
1 tablespoon prepared horseradish
¼ teaspoon pepper
1 tablespoon tomato purée
2kg (4lb) peeled prawns

Boil water in pan. Remove from heat and place tomatoes in the water for 5 minutes. Remove and skin tomatoes. (Discard water.) Chop tomatoes and mix with Tabasco, horseradish, pepper, and tomato purée in blender for 1 to 2 minutes to liquefy. Chill and serve with prawns.

Serves 4

PRAWNS WITH HOT SAUCE

½ teaspoon prepared horseradish
5 teaspoons dry mustard
5 teaspoons water
175-225g (6-8oz) peeled prawns

Mix horseradish, mustard, and water in small dish. Stir together thoroughly. Chill and serve with prawns.

Serves 1

LAMB WITH MINT SAUCE

8 tablespoons finely chopped fresh mint
¼ tablespoon sugar substitute
8 tablespoons vinegar
700g (1½lb) lamb (from any cut)

Mix mint, sugar substitute, and vinegar in small saucepan and cook over low heat until sugar substitute has dissolved. Chill overnight. Cook lamb your usual way for the type of cut. Pour mint sauce over individual servings to taste.

Serves 4

Potatoes and Rice

MELANIE'S MASHED POTATO SURPRISE

1 medium baking potato
2 tablespoons skimmed milk
½ teaspoon finely chopped onion
2 fresh mushrooms, finely chopped
½ teaspoon finely chopped fresh parsley
pepper to taste

Peel potato and boil for 30 minutes. Mash potato and slowly blend in milk. Add onion, mushrooms, and parsley. Add pepper to taste and serve. Add diet margarine only if specified in menu plan.

Serves 1

ROASTED CHIPS

1 medium baking potato

Cut *unpeeled* potato into eighths lengthwise. Place wedges on baking sheet and bake at 230°C (450°F) Gas 8 for 40 minutes. The chips will be browned and crispy on the outside and taste like a baked potato on the inside.

Serves 1

TWICE-BAKED POTATO

1 large baking potato
50g (2oz) cottage cheese
½ teaspoon chopped chives

Bake potato at 180°C (350°F) Gas 4 for 45 minutes. Cut potato in half and empty insides into bowl. Mix with cottage cheese and refill potato skin. Top with chives. Return to oven and bake at 180°C (350°F) Gas 4 for 20 minutes.

Serves 2 (½ potato each)

RICHARD'S POTATO SALAD

100g (4oz) diced cooked potatoes
1 hard-boiled egg (white only), diced
1 small celery stick, finely chopped
1 onion ring, finely chopped
1 tablespoon low-calorie onion or chive dressing
pepper to taste

Mix all ingredients together and serve.

Serves 1

POTATO CASSEROLE

1 medium potato
1 tablespoon low-fat natural yoghurt
1 tablespoon chopped onion
1 fresh mushroom, chopped
1 tablespoon chopped fresh parsley

Boil potato for 30 minutes. Peel and dice. Mix with yoghurt, onion, mushroom, and parsley. Place ingredients in small casserole dish and lightly brush with oil. Bake at 170°C (325°F) Gas 3 for 30 minutes or until hot and bubbly.

Serves 2

CURRIED RICE

100ml (4fl oz) chicken stock (see recipe, page 196)
100ml (4fl oz) water
½ teaspoon curry powder
75g (3oz) rice (uncooked)

Place chicken stock, water, and curry powder in saucepan and bring to a boil. Stir in rice. Turn heat to low and cover pan. Cook for 15 to 20 minutes. Serve 50g (2oz) portions (Low-cal menu plan).

Serves 3

FLAVOURED RICE

225ml (8 fl oz) water
75g (3oz) rice (uncooked)
2 tablespoons chopped fresh parsley
1 tablespoon diet margarine

Place water in saucepan and bring to a boil. Stir in rice and parsley. Turn heat to low and cover. Cook for 15 to 20 minutes. On serving, melt ⅓ tablespoon margarine over each portion.

Serves 3

Pasta and Pizza

VERMICELLI SCIACCA

225g (8oz) vermicelli
2 tablespoons diet margarine
100g (4oz) ricotta cheese
2 tablespoons chopped fresh parsley
2 tablespoons grated Parmesan cheese
freshly ground black pepper

Cook vermicelli *al dente*. Drain and place in warm bowl with 1 tablespoon melted margarine. Stir ricotta in saucepan with remaining tablespoon margarine, and heat until smooth, stirring continuously. Pour over vermicelli. Sprinkle with parsley, Parmesan cheese, and ground pepper. Toss all ingredients together. Serve 100g (4oz) per person.

Serves 3

MICHAEL'S FETTUCCINI ALFREDO

225g (8oz) fettuccini
1 teaspoon diet margarine
1 tablespoon skimmed milk
3 tablespoons low-fat natural yoghurt

1 egg white, hard-boiled
2 tablespoons grated Parmesan cheese
freshly ground black pepper

Cook fettuccini *al dente*. Place margarine in serving dish.
Add fettuccini and toss gently until margarine has mixed
with the noodles. In a separate small bowl, mix skimmed
milk and yoghurt until thoroughly blended. Add to
fettuccini and toss. Add egg white, grated cheese, and
pepper and toss once again.

Serves 3

SPAGHETTI WITH TOMATO SAUCE

3 cups skinned and chopped tomatoes
1 clove garlic, crushed
225g (8oz) chopped onion
2 tablespoons tomato purée
¼ teaspoon dried oregano
¼ teaspoon dried basil
1 bay leaf
¼ teaspoon ground pepper
225g (8oz) spaghetti

Place tomatoes in frying pan over medium heat. Add
garlic, onion, tomato purée, oregano, basil, bay leaf, and
pepper. Turn heat to low and cover. Simmer for 30 minutes, stirring occasionally. Cook spaghetti *al dente*. Remove bay leaf from sauce, pour over cooked spaghetti and
serve.

Serves 3

PIETRO'S PIZZA

4 egg whites
1 whole egg
50g (2oz) plain flour
½ teaspoon Italian seasoning
50ml (2 fl oz) tomato sauce
1 tablespoon grated Parmesan cheese

Mix egg whites, egg, flour, and Italian seasoning in a blender for 1 minute. Pour the mixture into a 30cm (12-inch) round tin that has been lightly brushed with oil. Bake at 180°C (350°F) Gas 4 for 12 minutes. Remove from oven and spread tomato sauce on top. Sprinkle with Parmesan cheese. Return to oven for another 5 to 8 minutes. Serves one person for an entrée, or ¼ pizza can serve as a metabo-meal – ½ pizza during Booster weeks.

Vegetables

LEMON BUTTER VEGETABLES

350g (12oz) green beans, broccoli, or asparagus
1½ tablespoons diet margarine
½ teaspoon lemon juice
½ teaspoon chopped fresh parsley

Steam or boil vegetables until tender, then drain. While cooking vegetables mix margarine, lemon juice, and parsley in small saucepan. Heat at medium temperature for 5 minutes. Pour over vegetables and serve.

Serves 3

CARROTS WITH MINT

225g (8oz) sliced carrots
½ teaspoon finely chopped fresh mint

Steam or boil carrots until tender. Drain off water and serve. Sprinkle mint over each serving.

Serves 2

HOT VEGETABLE PLATTER

100g (4oz) broccoli
100g (4oz) cauliflower
100g (4oz) carrots
100g (4oz) green beans
50g (2oz) mushrooms
3 spring onions
3 tablespoons diet dressing (Italian or herbal type)
1 tablespoon grated Parmesan cheese

Steam broccoli, cauliflower, carrots, and green beans until tender yet slightly crispy. Sauté mushrooms and onions in dressing until soft. Combine all cooked ingredients, and toss. Place in casserole dish and sprinkle with Parmesan cheese. Bake for 10 minutes at 200°C (400°F) Gas 6. Serve as a luncheon dish with fruit for dessert.

Serves 1

STEWED TOMATOES

225g (8oz) skinned and chopped tomatoes
1 tablespoon chopped onion
1 tablespoon chopped green pepper
¼ teaspoon dried oregano

¼ teaspoon dried basil
¼ teaspoon artificial sweetener

Mix all ingredients in saucepan with 2 tablespoons water. Cover and simmer over low heat for 20 minutes.

Serves 2

MARROW CASSEROLE

175g (6oz) sliced marrow
1 tablespoon chopped onion
2 tablespoons cottage cheese
¼ teaspoon caraway seeds
freshly ground black pepper
1 teaspoon grated Parmesan cheese

Steam or boil marrow and onion until tender. (Do not overcook.) Drain and mix in cottage cheese, caraway seeds, and pepper. Place in baking dish and sprinkle top with Parmesan cheese. Bake at 180°C (350°F) Gas 4 for 30 minutes.

Serves 2

Salads, Dressings, and Dips

ALICE'S CHICKEN SALAD

700g (1½lb) diced cooked chicken (4 breasts)
100g (4oz) chopped celery
1 small apple, chopped
2 tablespoons chopped onion
100g (4oz) cottage cheese
1 teaspoon skimmed milk
pepper

Mix chicken, celery, apple, and onion in large mixing bowl. In a blender mix cottage cheese and skimmed milk. Blend for 2 minutes on high speed. Add to chicken mixture. Season to taste. Serve on a lettuce leaf or in a sandwich.

Serves 4

COLD CRAB SALAD

75g (3oz) fresh shredded cabbage
75g (3oz) cooked crabmeat
¼ apple, diced
½ small celery stalk, finely chopped
½ tablespoon melted diet margarine

Toss all ingredients together and chill. Serve over lettuce or stuffed into a tomato.

Serves 1

TOMATO AND CUCUMBER SALAD

1 medium tomato
6 thin cucumber slices
fresh watercress sprigs
1 tablespoon diet Italian dressing

Cut tomato in sixths from top almost through to the bottom. Tuck cucumber slices and watercress sprigs into the slits. Top with dressing. Serve with fruit for lunch.

Serves 1

SPINACH SALAD

75g (3oz) chopped fresh spinach
25g (1oz) sliced fresh mushrooms
½ onion, sliced into rings
1 medium hard-boiled egg, sliced
2 tablespoons diet dressing of choice
pepper to taste

Toss all ingredients together in large bowl and serve.

Serves 1

TUNA SALAD

75g (3oz) tuna fish (water-packed)
1 tablespoon chopped celery stalk
1 pinch thyme
1 tablespoon diet salad dressing (mayonnaise type)

Mix all ingredients in mixing bowl. Serve on lettuce leaf or in sandwich.

Serves 1

CREAMY THICK DRESSING

50g (2oz) cottage cheese
100ml (4 fl oz) buttermilk or low-fat natural yoghurt
¼ teaspoon dill weed
2 teaspoons chopped parsley
1½ teaspoons minced onion
1 teaspoon dry mustard
Tabasco sauce to taste

Mix all ingredients thoroughly in blender. Chill in refrigerator before serving. Serve 2 to 3 tablespoons over salad.

CURRIED DRESSING

225ml (8 fl oz) natural yoghurt
½ tablespoon dry mustard
½ teaspoon curry powder
1 tablespoon finely chopped parsley

Mix all ingredients thoroughly in blender. Chill in refrigerator before serving. Serve 2 to 3 tablespoons over salad.

TOMATO HERB DRESSING

300ml (½pint) tinned tomato soup
1 tablespoon tarragon vinegar
½ teaspoon dill
½ teaspoon basil
1 teaspoon Worcestershire sauce

Mix all ingredients thoroughly in blender. Chill in refrigerator before serving. Serve 2 to 3 tablespoons over salad.

HERB DIP

1 tablespoon skimmed milk
2 tablespoons cottage cheese
2 tablespoons ricotta cheese
1 teaspoon parsley
¼ teaspoon paprika
¼ teaspoon lemon juice

¼ teaspoon dill weed
¼ teaspoon Worcestershire sauce
½ teaspoon finely chopped onion
6 drops Tabasco sauce

Place all ingredients in blender and mix until smooth.
Chill and serve with raw vegetables.

Fruit

FRUIT AMBROSIA

½ apple, finely chopped
½ orange, finely chopped
½ grapefruit, finely chopped
8 seedless grapes
⅛ honeydew melon, finely chopped
¼ cantaloupe, finely chopped
shredded coconut

Combine fruit ingredients in mixing bowl and chill.
Sprinkle servings lightly with coconut.

Serves 2 metabo-meals or 5 desserts with dinner

GRAPEFRUIT JELLY

1 envelope gelatine
2 whole grapefruit (juice only)
2 tablespoons freshly squeezed lemon juice
4 tablespoons freshly squeezed orange juice
½ tablespoon sugar substitute

Combine gelatine and 3 tablespoons grapefruit juice in
bowl. Boil 225ml (8 fl oz) grapefruit juice in saucepan.

Slowly stir gelatine mixture into the boiled grapefruit juice. Stir in lemon juice, orange juice, and sugar substitute. Chill for several hours.

Serves 4

LOW-CAL BAKED APPLE

1 medium apple
½ teaspoon nutmeg
1 teaspoon brown sugar substitute

Core and halve apple. Mix nutmeg with brown sugar substitute. Sprinkle over apple and bake for 30 minutes at 180°C (350°F) Gas 4. Baste the apple halves with the liquid while baking. Sprinkle top with extra nutmeg before serving.

Serves 2

PURDY'S PEARS

1 medium pear
½ teaspoon cinnamon
1 teaspoon brown sugar substitute

Core and halve pear. Mix cinnamon with brown sugar substitute. Sprinkle over pear halves and bake for 30 minutes at 180°C (350°F) Gas 4. Sprinkle top with extra cinnamon before serving.

Serves 2

JESSIE MAE'S STRAWBERRY SURPRISE

450ml (¾pint) water
1 packet jelly
275g (10oz) sliced strawberries

Add 225ml (8 fl oz) boiling water to 1 envelope of
gelatine. Stir until dissolved. Add 225ml (8 fl oz) water.
Chill and let gelatine firm slightly. Add strawberries. Continue to chill until set.

Serves 4

21
A Final Word

Now that you know about the Hilton Head Metabolism Diet, get started right away. A new slim life awaits you. Can you imagine – a new body and a new metabolism. You've been waiting for the Hilton Head Metabolism Diet all your life, and here it is. Believe me, dieting will never be the same.

You must promise me two things. First, you must *never ever* go on any other diet again. The Hilton Head Metabolism Diet is the *only* way to accomplish your goal. So forget everything you've learned about dieting. And never listen to friends and their theories of dieting. Join the thousands of converts to the Hilton Head Metabolism Diet. It's the *only* way to make sure you're slim for ever. It's the *only* diet that will finally allow you to eat like a normal person, like a slim person.

The second promise you must make is to follow my entire plan exactly as I have described it. *You must*

- Start on the Low-cal menu plan.

- Switch to the Booster menus every third week.

- Eat four meals every day.

- Use my Calorie Burners after at least two meals every day.

- As you lose weight, add my Muscle Firmers three days a week.

- Switch to Reentry menus to get you ready for Maintenance.

- Weigh and take your measurements on a regular basis to see how you're doing.

Don't leave out any of these basic elements. If you follow my plan to the letter, you'll succeed. You must not modify the plan, or it won't work for you. Suppose your doctor gave you three pills to cure you of a life-threatening disease. Would you take only one of them? Of course not. Well, your metabolic suppression is like a disease, and I'm giving you the cure – the only cure.

Before you know it, you'll look and feel totally different. You'll have a slim figure, a firm body, an efficient metabolism, and a new outlook on life. And best of all, your dieting days will be over for ever.

Index